MEDIUM SECURE PSYCHIATRIC PRO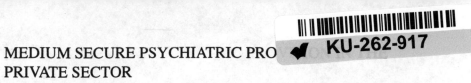
PRIVATE SECTOR

MEDIUM SECURE PSYCHIATRIC PROVISION IN THE
PRIVATE SECTOR

For Gemma and Christopher

Medium Secure Psychiatric Provision in the Private Sector

KATRINA R. MOSS

Ashgate

Aldershot • Brookfield USA • Singapore • Sydney

Published by
Ashgate Publishing Ltd
Gower House
Croft Road
Aldershot
Hants GU11 3HR
England

Ashgate Publishing Company
Old Post Road
Brookfield
Vermont 05036
USA

British Library Cataloguing in Publication Data
Moss, Katrina R.
    Medium secure psychiatric provision in the private sector
    1.Mental health services - Great Britain 2.Mental health
    services - United States 3.Health facilities, Propietary -
    Great Britain 4.Health facilities, Proprietary - United
    States
    I. Title
    362.2'1'0941

Library of Congress Catalog Card Number: 98-73023

ISBN 1 84014 310 X

Printed and bound by Athenaeum Press, Ltd.,
Gateshead, Tyne & Wear.

Contents

List of Tables

Preface

The policy of privatisation has been widely discussed over a number of years since its inception, primarily in the United States and its subsequent travel across the Atlantic to the United Kingdom. In both jurisdictions the ideology has been advocated by proponents of libertarian socioeconomic policies and in Britain has received the long-standing commitment of the Conservatives. Notwithstanding this, relatively little attention has been paid to the privatisation of psychiatric care in the United Kingdom. As such, this is a neglected field of study.

Private medical care has been, and remains, a salient feature on the health care landscape. It is significant not only in terms of policy, as a great deal of political importance has been and continues to be attached to it, but also in terms of medicine and concentrates on specific specialties much of the time. It is one of these specialties – medium secure independent psychiatric provision – with which this study will seek to deal. In doing so it will address the contribution currently being made to the existing public service by the recently introduced private provision.

Acknowledgments

I would like to thank the following people for their help in making the completion of this book possible.

First I would like to thank Professor Ken Pease for supervising this project and for seeing the thesis on which it is based through to its completion in spite of his move from Manchester to Huddersfield. Although he will not like me saying all these things, (because in spite of his impressive reputation he is a truly modest and self-effacing person) I would still like to thank him for his infinite wisdom, his sound, down-to-earth advice and his endless encouragement and humour.

Thanks must also go to Wendy Buck for her support at the start of this project and for spending so much of her time with me and the SPSS data entry system.

I would like to thank Staffordshire University Law School for their support and most important for allowing me the study leave necessary to complete it, without which it would have been an impossible task.

Thanks also to the staff and patients of Stockton Hall, York, the Hutton Unit, Middlesbrough and the Norvic Clinic, Norwich. In particular to Dr Chris Green who organised my fieldwork at all of these facilities and who put me up (or was it put up with me?) during my stint at the Hutton.

I would like to thank the Department of Social Policy at the University of Manchester for keeping in touch with me throughout the past four years. As a part-time student I have very much appreciated this. I would also like to thank Paul Wilding and Ian Gough who gave me so much encouragement and lent me so many books (all of which I have returned, I hasten to add).

Many thanks to my husband Paul for helping me to collect data at Middlesbrough and Norwich and for explaining chi-square to me! I count myself truly fortunate, although I probably don't ever say it, to have such a wonderful husband.

Thanks also go of course to my Mum and Dad for their interest, encouragement and much appreciated help with the children. Parents of all people often receive the least thanks when they actually deserve the most, so I would like to put the record straight and say thank you for your endless support of my educational endeavours over many many years. I could not have done any of this if it were not for both of you. Thanks also for proving time and time again what a great institution grandparents are.

Finally, I want to mention and thank sincerely all the staff at the North Staffs Oral Surgery Department, but most particularly my hero of the NHS, Consultant Surgeon Peter Leopard, without whose knowledge and expertise I simply would not have been around to finish this. Thank you.

Introduction

Chapter 1 focuses on the meaning of the term privatisation, its origins and development in the United States and the United Kingdom, the philosophical and economic background to this and the policy issues surrounding its implementation.

Chapter 2 reviews the range of attitudes surrounding the policy implications of privatisation within the criminal justice system. Specifically it considers the privatisation of prisons in the United States and the United Kingdom, tracing this development and the emotional debate which has surrounded its implementation.

Chapter 3 provides a review of the most current literature on the provision of private psychiatric care in the United States and the United Kingdom. This provides insight into the prevalence of, attitudes to and success of private health care and a comparison of the concerns voiced in relation to its implementation. It identifies the issues of access, profit, quality and community needs as being areas of concern in the provision of private psychiatric care and explains the reasons for the subsequent focus of this study on access to that care in both the public and private sectors.

Chapter 4 provides an explanation of the legal and medical issues involved in the provision of mental health care, its regulation by the Mental Health Act 1983 and how this legislation deals with persons who are deemed to require psychiatric care in conditions of security. It also explains the procedures necessary for sectioning under the Mental Health Act and the passage into secure care of those deemed by the law to require it.

Chapter 5 traces the development of public sector medium secure regional psychiatric provision, the introduction of the Regional Secure Unit and the place which such units occupy in the Mental Health System. It includes an empirical study of admissions and discharges to two public sector Regional Secure Units during the period 1989 to 1992 and seeks to address the issue of access to psychiatric care in the public sector.

Chapter 6 discusses the advent of independent medium secure psychiatric care and considers how this sort of provision fits into the national picture of medium secure psychiatric care. It includes an empirical study of admissions

1

and discharges to an independent medium secure psychiatric hospital between 1989 and 1992 and illustrates some variations in access to private psychiatric care compared to that provided by the public sector.

Chapter 7 considers a cohort of 59 patients identified in chapter 6 as having been admitted to private psychiatric care after having been classified as unmanageable in their parent district. This detailed account of patient characteristics and how they came to be in private secure care, rather than that provided by their home district, gives a useful insight into an aspect of the variation in access which exists in relation to public and private sector medium secure psychiatric care and which was outlined in chapter 6.

Chapter 8 seeks to review the findings of the studies described in chapters 5, 6 and 7. It outlines the differences existing in relation to patient access to public and private psychiatric care and the motivating forces which may explain these variations. In doing so it suggests that an essentially pluralistic culture of medium secure psychiatric provision has become the hallmark of the '90s in this sphere, and that this has occurred rather more by accident than design.

1 Privatisation, the General Issues

This study seeks to address the contribution being made by the private sector to the provision of medium secure psychiatric care in England and Wales. In order to provide a background for this, it is necessary to illustrate the origins and development of privatisation first in the United States, where the most recent trends originated and subsequently in the United Kingdom. This chapter considers the definition of the term privatisation, the philosophical and theoretical aspects of the current resurgence of privatisation and the policy issues which have been raised regarding its general implementation.

Defining Privatisation

The concept of privatisation is not new and can be found in the work of the philosopher and economist Adam Smith as early as 1762. The term 'privatisation' however, *is* relatively new and can be broadly defined as meaning the transfer of a function or an activity from the public sector to the private. Alternatively, according to Adam et al. (1992, p. 6), it could be used to describe:

> an array of actions designed to broaden the scope of private sector activity, or the assimilation by the public sector, of efficiency-enhancing techniques generally employed by the private sector.

Privatisation is a process or an approach and essentially no definition can wholly encompass something which may have different interpretations and applications. This is because privatisation can occur in a number of different ways. First, it is possible to transfer a publicly owned asset (by sale) to the private sector completely and this may entail the government having no further responsibility from this point. This type of privatisation is fairly straightforward from the point of view of understanding what it means but it can be the most difficult to achieve. Second, it is possible for the state to retain partial ownership of a public asset, but to sell parts to other buyers usually by public flotation on the stock market. In this way the government can retain a majority share if this is desirable but the service is actually managed privately. Another alternative is to lease or franchise assets. This means that whilst ownership remains with the government (i.e. it is still a state owned enterprise or SOE), the management of the asset is in the private sector.

In general terms to privatise is to render private. It is a withdrawal of the state from the production of goods and services and its roots can be found in the concept of the free market and historically, the liberal, socioeconomic ideologies of the Enlightenment. These ideas are now discussed.

Philosophical and Theoretical Backgrounds to Privatisation

According to Johnson (1988, p. 60):

> [a]ll privatisations are motivated to some extent by the ideological belief that the State's role in the economy should be diminished and that of the private sector increased.

This is essentially the idea of promoting what are called 'laissez-faire economics', but where do these ideologies have their roots?

Shichor (1995) describes the Enlightenment as being the intellectual and sociocultural basis of modern Western civilisation with the 'classical liberal' approach reflected in the work of writers such as Thomas Hobbes (1588–1679), John Locke (1632–1704) and Adam Smith (1723–1790). In Hobbes' *Leviathan*, the nature of the state was integral and the idea of the 'social contract' was expounded whereby citizens were seen to accept the establishment of the commonwealth as a means of protecting their personal rights. Locke also believed that the role of the state was to provide protection and this explained people's wish to belong to the civilised society. Perhaps the most influential was Adam Smith's *The Wealth of Nations* in which he pioneered economic liberalism, promoting the idea of free trade and free competition as being the most effective ways of ensuring successful economic policy. According to Shichor (1995, pp. 4–5) '[H]e argued that free competition among private enterprises would result in greater income for everyone' and that 'if everyone would be allowed to follow free economic action, the competing individual interests, without any state intervention, would produce the most real wealth and happiness among the nations'.

Smith's main idea was the system of 'natural liberty'. By this he meant that it was right to strive for a competitive market where trade is free and takes place within the rule of law. In this market place the consumer was all-important and the market served the consumer within a system of self-regulation. For instance, the dishonest trader would be undercut by other traders and find his profits falling as would the trader who charges excessive prices for goods. This Smith called the 'Invisible Hand'. He believed that in the free market place, two factors were of prime importance. These were first the element of competition and second that of liberty.

In respect of competition, Smith believed that this idea was rooted in the concept of power. He believed that if producers were too powerful, they would overcharge for goods and services which may also be of inferior quality. Here the concept of competition was very powerful because it acted to restrain this behaviour. In this sense he felt that competition brought about a close relationship between economic power and benefit to the consumers of goods and services.

In terms of liberty, for libertarians like Smith, economic freedom would be a prerequisite for political freedom. According to Friedman (1980, p. 223):

> [t]hat is the basic difference between the market and a political agency. You are free to choose. There is no policeman to take your money out of your pocket to pay for something you do not want or to make you do something you do not want to do.

In this way the market is seen as a democratic system of persuasion.

This is essentially the explanation for liberal political theory, which although it may be elaborated on, is a fairly simple mechanism and one which has provided the basis for moves both in the United States and United Kingdom towards State deregulation over the past 15–20 years. It is these ideas which have been the most influential in terms of American socioeconomic ideology. They were strongly reinforced during the 1970s and 1980s when the Americans, concerned about the decline in American economic power, the rise in crime and fresh from their involvement in the Vietnam War, began to look to politically conservative ideals as a means of resolving their social and economic problems. In his book *Privatising the Public Sector*, Savas takes up this point saying that by the mid-1970s the American people had almost totally lost faith in government, the majority believing that it had too much power. The effect on the social contract between the government and the people, was that they had, in their minds and hearts, withdrawn their consent. This, he says, was one of the major reasons for the election of Ronald Reagan as president. His promise to limit the size of federal government was seen as a reflection of the widespread opposition to the role successive United States governments had so far taken. As a critic of 'big government', Savas explains its growth, why shrinking it is a good idea and suggests a number of ways of achieving this.

Savas contends that there are strong pressures for government to grow. It can be as a response to public demand, because service producers want to supply more services or as a consequence of inefficiency. He suggests (1982, p. 25) that:

> [i]f unchecked, these factors would lead to an unstable and uncontrollable spiral of continued growth: the bigger the Government, the greater the force for even bigger Government ... The forecast seems ominous: Sooner or later everyone will be working for the Government.

He claims that the result of this is that (1982, p. 26):

> [v]oters reject spending proposals, elect more frugal officials and flee from high-tax jurisdiction. President Carter was elected in part because of his *non*-Washington background; President Reagan was elected in great measure because of his *anti*-Washington stance: Get the government off the backs of the people.

As a result he says that the thing to strive for is a more limited and sensible role for government and to find alternative ways of providing services. Some of the examples he uses are franchises, grants and vouchers and I select these from the number that he gives because they are some of the more familiar ones to us in the United Kingdom.

Franchises can be either exclusive or nonexclusive. In an exclusive franchise the government awards monopoly privileges to a private firm to supply a particular service, the price usually being regulated by the government. In a nonexclusive (sometimes called multiple) franchise a number of firms can supply the service. In both situations, the government is the arranger and the private firm the producer and the consumer pays the producer. Examples of services which Savas says can be most suitably franchised are cable television, electricity, water and gas.

Grants and vouchers are methods of providing services where the consumption of the particular product is to be encouraged. In the grant system, the producer is a private firm, the government and the consumer can be involved as arrangers and both the government and the consumer make payments to the producer. Under this system, a subsidy is given to the producer by the government perhaps by a tax-exempt grant, or more usually by a direct grant of money, in an effort to reduce the price of certain goods or services and thus make them more affordable to the average consumer. Familiar examples of this system would be universities as beneficiaries of grants together with the more recent example of cultural and artistic institutions such as symphony orchestras and opera companies.

Vouchers are similarly a means of encouraging the consumer in respect of certain goods and services, but differ from the grant system in that vouchers subsidise the consumer, not the producer and so allow the consumer an element of free choice in the market place. One example which most people would be familiar with would be food vouchers and in the United States, because they do not have a National Health Service like our own, a common example of this system would be vouchers for medical care. These take the form of what are known in the United States as Medicaid or Medicare enrolment cards. In the United Kingdom, our most recent brush with the voucher system has been in connection with vouchers for the provision of preschool nursery education. These are just a few examples.

Using methods such as these, it is possible to limit the size and scope of government which is obviously biggest when there are a lot of public services and smallest when systems of franchise are used, together with grants and vouchers, which require some government expenditure, but less than an alternative public sector based system.

Savas claims (1982, p. 89) that of all the alternatives which work to limit the growth of government:

> [t]he most promising ones in this respect ... are primarily the ones that can be called private-sector alternatives: market, contract, franchise, voucher and grant arrangements. In each of these, the private sector is the producer, in contrast to governmental and intergovernmental arrangements, in which Government is the producer.

Since moves have been made once more, in the United States and the United Kingdom towards greater private involvement in many traditionally public services, it is making a choice between these two – public or private – and the argument over which is best and for whom, that has sparked off a lengthy and often emotional debate between the opponents and supporters of privatisation. For the record and for the sake of equity, it is worth noting what have been generally regarded as the main arguments for and against this approach. It has been argued that:

1   contracting is more efficient because:

   a) it harnesses competitive forces and brings the pressure of the market place to bear on inefficient producers;
   b) it permits better management, free of overtly political organisations;
   c) the costs and benefits of managerial decisions are felt more directly by the decision maker, whose own rewards are directly at stake;

2   contracting makes it possible for government to take advantage of specialised skills ... and overcome obsolete salary limitations and antiquated civil service restrictions;

3   it allows flexibility in adjusting the size of a programme in response to changing demand or fund availability;

4   it permits a quicker response to new needs and facilitates experimentation in new programmes;

5   it is a way of avoiding large capital outlays, spreading costs over a time at a relatively constant and predictable level;

6   it permits economies of scale regardless of the scale of the government entity involved;

7   contracting a portion of the work offers a yardstick for comparison: the cost of the service is highly visible in the price of the contract, unlike most government services;

8   it can reduce dependence on a single supplier (a government monopoly) and so lessens the vulnerability of the service to strikes, slowdowns and inept leadership;

9   it limits the size of government, at least in terms of the number of employees.

   On the other side of the coin, there are also many reasons why privatisation is not thought to be such a good idea. For instance, it has been argued that:

1   contracting is ultimately more expensive because of:

a) corruption;
b) high profits;
c) the cost of layoffs and unemployment for government workers;
d) the shortage of qualified suppliers and therefore the lack of competition;
e) the cost of managing the contract and monitoring contractor performance;
f) the low marginal cost of expanding government service;
g) cost-plus-fixed-fee provisions in some contracts, which provide no incentive for efficiency;
h) the absence of effective competition in 'follow-on' contracts, which are commonplace;

2 contracting nullifies the basic principle of merit employment and subverts laws regarding veterans' preference in government employment; it is demoralizing to employees, deprives government of the skills it needs in-house and therefore is fundamentally debilitating of government capability;

3 contracting limits the flexibility of government in responding to emergencies;

4 it fosters an undesirable dependence on contractors and leaves the public vulnerable to strikes and slowdowns by contractor personnel and to bankruptcy of the firm;

5 it depends on adequately written contracts, which are difficult to draw up and as a result there is a loss of government accountability and control;

6 it limits the opportunity to realise economies of scale;

7 entrusting some services to private organisations might increase their political power to such an extent that there would be a general loss of independence for other public and private entities;

8 contracting causes a loss of autonomy of the contractor and therefore decreases the latter's effectiveness in the long run by muting its role as critic and social conscience (reproduced from Savas, 1982, pp. 89–91).

Pertinent also to this study is the argument in the corrections and police context about threatening the state monopoly on violence. These, broadly speaking, are the claims and counter claims in respect of any move towards greater privatisation. Essentially however, it cannot really be that simple. Whilst accepting that today's economy is much more mixed than it has been for some significant time, Wilding (1989) suggests that in the United Kingdom the approach has not yet been implemented fully enough to assess its success or failure as a policy. His concern is that some of the justifications for it have been too vague and that the real complexities of the issue have not yet been fully explored. His suggestion is that there are five areas where it is possible to look behind the approach to the real significance of the policies which have been pursued by the British government. Wilding's first concern is that the move from public to private provision is not necessarily the correct solution to the problem of the provision of efficient, effective and acceptable services. He suggests (1989, p. 28) that:

> [t]he Government's seeming belief that the solution to current doubts and ills is to move from public to private provision bypasses the debate which could and should be taking place about whether and when public provision has advantages, and whether and when private provision should be favoured ...

Second, he suggests that the move to greater privatisation means the state's role is reduced and becomes less clear. There is a 'blurring' of the distinction between the public and the private without having had a real discussion regarding the choices.

Third, Wilding suggests (1989, p. 28) that

> privatisation affects attitudes to welfare. To argue for private provision of services is to make an implicit statement about the individual nature of need and responsibility.

He indicates that whilst it might well be possible to meet certain needs by private provision, which could not have been so met prior to 1948, this does not necessarily mean that the reasons to provide it collectively no longer exist. Accepting that the move to privatisation is in part a reflection of changes in society, he cautions that 'its impact needs very careful assessment' (1989, p. 29).

Fourth, Wilding warns that privatisation is capable of creating social division – for instance between people who have private pensions (who will obviously be better off) and those who do not.

He also suggests that it affects other areas such as the health service and the growth of private medicine, possibly making those who can afford private medical insurance complacent as to ensuring the continued provision of the NHS for those who are and will remain dependent on it.

Finally, he indicates that privatisation is, of course, a significant economic strategy in terms of raising capital and reducing taxes which has been a major goal of the Conservatives since 1979.

Undoubtedly, as Wilding suggests, the concept of privatisation *is* rooted in certain beliefs as has already been indicated in this chapter. It may well be the case that certain services can be provided efficiently and effectively by the private sector, but the same could also be said of the public sector. In order to make the right choices it is necessary to be aware of all the advantages and disadvantages of each system of provision and that according to Wilding (1989, p. 30) 'the supporters and opponents of privatisation ... should be pressed to develop the arguments and clarify the issues'.

The next section looks briefly at the recent trend in commitment to privatisation in the United States and in more detail at its subsequent resurgence in the United Kingdom.

Privatisation in the United States

The origins of privatisation in its current form lie in the eighteenth century with the ideas embodied in Adam Smith's *The Wealth of Nations* and Thomas Jefferson's Declaration of Independence. Both were singularly influential in terms of American socioeconomic ideas and have since been referred to by Milton Friedman (1980) as the ideas which set in motion what he terms the economic and political miracle of America resulting in laissez-faire economics and the free market. According to Friedman (1980, pp. 2–3);

> [e]conomic freedom is an essential requisite for political freedom. By enabling people to cooperate with one another without coercion or central direction, it reduces the area over which political power is exercised. In addition, by dispersing power, the free market provides an offset to whatever concentration of political power may arise. The combination of economic and political power in the same hands is a sure recipe for tyranny.

Over time these ideas have led to what could be termed a negative American approach to public management which was reinforced from the 1970s onwards. From this time the aversion to 'big' government grew in the United States and the move towards deregulation gained impetus during the Reagan administration which began to implement classical-liberal socioeconomic ideas. The result of this was that during this time a large-scale deregulation took place, sparking off the naming of this era, amongst those opposed to the policies, as the 'dismantling of America'. Instrumental in achieving these policies were the recommendations of the Grace Commission which strongly urged the use of initiatives for reaching privatisation goals and the implementation of Proposition 13 which aimed to curb state and local expenditure. Fraser and Wilson (1988, p. 155) emphasise how committed the Reagan administration was to this aim from the outset, by citing an excerpt from the President's inaugural speech on 20 January 1981 where he promised to 'check and reverse the growth of government which shows signs of having grown beyond the consent of the governed'.

It could be argued that the processes implemented to achieve this subsequently did not come as much of a shock to the Americans in comparison to similar moves later made in the United Kingdom. This was probably because in the United States, there was already a tradition that the federal government did not really involve itself in the manufacture or supply of goods and services, with the exception of some areas of social welfare and defence. The main problem for the Reagan administration was the swollen budget deficit which it determined to reduce by 1991. As a result, a number of measures were implemented. These included the enactment of the Emergency Deficit Control Bill in 1985 which incorporated the 'Gramm-Rudman Amendment' stipulating the move towards a balanced budget to be achieved by 1991. It was after this that the President announced the intention to privatise some federal assets and this was passed by Congress in 1986. Some of the assets recommended for this by the Commission on Privatisation 1987, chaired by David Linowes, were postal operations, prisons, and railways. A school voucher system for parents to purchase their children's education was also discussed. One example of the significant moves towards privatisation which subsequently occurred in the United States was the sale of the Consolidated Rail Corporation (Conrail). Under Elizabeth Dole the (then) transport secretary, this was offered for sale publicly in 1987 and was estimated to have made $1.9 billion for the United States government. Commenting on this, Fraser and Wilson (1988, p. 157) quote Elizabeth Dole as having said 'we have succeeded in the largest privatisation in American history, and this success should break ground for more privatisations to come'.

Without doubt, the trend towards privatisation as the solution to a number of economic ills in the United States, was influential upon the British government under Mrs Thatcher. She and President Reagan shared many ideals and a mutual political respect. It is not surprising therefore, that these ideas began to cross the Atlantic, sparking a renewed interest in privatisation as an approach with which the Conservatives could identify, both ideologically and economically. The following section looks at the rise of this trend in the United Kingdom.

Privatisation in the United Kingdom

Although it was certainly the case that the American experience influenced the Conservatives, this was part of a process already under way when they formed a government in 1979. Veljanovski (1988, p. 24) suggests that '[the] intellectual offensive of what is called the New Right predates the rise of Mrs Thatcher' and that after the defeat of the Heath government there was a substantial reworking of the Conservative Party philosophy led by Mrs Thatcher and Sir Keith Joseph. At this time the Centre for Policy Studies was set up, as was the Institute for Economic Affairs and these provided the intellectual basis for the subsequent economic policies of the party and what has since been termed the move to 'New Conservatism'.

This move represented a departure from the traditions of Tory paternalism and is connected to liberal political theory which has already been discussed in this chapter. Feeling that the party lacked a coherent economic theory, essentially distinct from that of Labour, the Conservatives began to move towards the more intellectual, radical and confrontational ideas of capitalism. This encompassed individualism, the importance of the profit motive and the entrepreneur, and aggressive advocacy of private enterprise and the market. Although it is possible to suggest that such policies are based solely upon political ideals, it is more realistic to attribute this move to a combination of ideas, circumstances and opportunity. An explanation of how the issue of privatisation became connected with all this is suggested by Veljanovski (1988, p. 32) who contends;

> [t]he important implication of this approach is that privatisation occurred not because someone in the Conservative Party thought it was an intellectually coherent and attractive idea or because Mrs Thatcher was ideologically committed and determined to see it become a reality. Privatisation has occurred because within the economic and political forces operating in the 1980s it was the best way to achieve the Government's objective of reducing the role of the state in the economy.

It is possible to say, therefore, that privatisation was an idea which blended in with the Conservative Party's traditional support of private property, private enterprise and its disillusionment with the nationalised industries. At the same time it believed that privatisation could improve industrial performance and gave the following as its major objectives:

- the reduction of government involvement in decision-making of industry;

- to permit industry to raise funds from the capital market on commercial terms and without government guarantee;

- to raise revenue and reduce the public sector borrowing requirement (PSBR);

- to promote wide share ownership;

- to create an enterprise culture;

- to encourage workers' share ownership in their companies;

- to increase competition and efficiency;

- to replace ownership and financial controls with a more effective system of economic regulation designed to ensure that benefits of greater efficiency are passed on to consumers (reproduced from Veljanovski, 1988, p. 8).

It was on this basis that between 1979 and 1983, the government made plans to privatise a number of public enterprises which included Amersham International and British Rail Hotels, although these involved only the partial transfer of ownership. Outright sales were made of some of the subsidiaries of the National Enterprise Board, including Ferranti and International Computers. Over this four year period, approximately £1.4 billion was raised by the sale of public companies. This trend continued in their second term of office during which British Telecom was sold for almost £4 billion and British Gas for over £5 billion. These and other sales which have taken place since have resulted in reducing the government's involvement in production in the economy by more than a half and has radically changed the nature of government involvement and control over the previously nationalised sector. It has also produced the rise of the regulatory agency as a result, perhaps the most well known of which are the Office of Fair Trading and the Monopolies and Mergers Commission. Other specific agencies have also been introduced to regulate newly privatised industries, amongst others, OFTEL, OFWAT and OFGAS.

The privatisation policy therefore has been an ongoing feature of the Conservative Party's terms in government since 1979. During this time, it has been, and continues to be hotly debated and a number of major criticisms have emerged. First, it has been said that there has been no real coherent strategy or plan to the implementation of the policy. Second, that it has been based mainly on financial grounds in the sense that it raises money for the Treasury and can therefore assist with tax cuts and reducing public expenditure. Third, it has been claimed that flotations have been badly handled and shares undervalued with the result that a minority of individuals have made a fortune at the expense of the taxpayer and that other methods of sale should therefore have been employed. Finally it has been argued that the government has failed properly to analyse the effects and consequences of the policy.

There have also been responses to these criticisms. It is probably fair to say that its objectives have evolved over the years and this, in part, is what has kept the debate ongoing.

In the early 1980s the objectives of privatisation were most probably rooted in the largely ideological desire of the Conservatives to subject the nationalised industries to the competitive forces of the market place. Later on, privatisation appears to have taken on board more specific objectives. These have been outlined as moves to increase competition and efficiency and to create wider share ownership, which, it has been claimed, have been carried out by a large number of different methods. However, these objectives have always been criticised as being mere excuses for what opponents have felt are the real reasons for privatising. Supporters have also claimed in response to criticisms that the goals have not simply been financial, but that there have been important political dimensions to the sale of public assets. It has increased share ownership, fostered competition and has played an important role in changing people's attitudes in a society which has traditionally harboured anti-enterprise values. Therefore, it is claimed that if more people have an involvement in the performance of companies, they will become more politically aware, and that this is beneficial.

Discussion

Privatisation has been, and continues to be a policy of a overtly political nature. This makes it doubly difficult to assess the claims and counter claims made by its supporters and opponents and truly to evaluate it as it now exists. It is a complex policy which has involved more than any definition of the term could possibly convey. As Veljanovski suggests (1988, p. 19):

> [a] simple change of ownership does not of itself solve all the problems which have plagued the nationalised industries and which were responsible for their poor performance. Many remain, and must be tackled by new, regulatory techniques administered by independent authorities. But, and this is a crucial point, privatisation is more than a change in ownership from the Government to a small number of private individuals and institutions. It is a complex change in the objectives, property rights and business environment of each firm, and – in the case of the utility industries – a change in the system of controls they face and in their relationship with the Government. This brings us to the central point – the need to evaluate policy as it exists.

In spite of the high political profile privatisation has had in the United Kingdom during the last 16 or so years, its implementation and effects over this time require further examination. Outside the nationalised industries moves to privatise other specific areas such as criminal justice and health care provide opportunities for this type of investigation in relatively neglected fields. This study seeks to evaluate the move towards privatisation in one specific sphere, that of psychiatric care. In order to provide a basis for this, the next chapter seeks to review the range of attitudes surrounding the implementation of this policy in one related area – that of the criminal justice system – in particular the moves towards the privatisation of prisons in the United States and the United Kingdom. This development and the emotional debate which has surrounded it are examined.

2 Privatisation and the Criminal Justice System

Chapter 1 focused on the general origins and development of privatisation in the United States and the United Kingdom. It illustrated that current interest in privatisation originated in the work of economists such as Milton Friedman and Adam Smith, whose work advocated the benefits of privatisation and the free market as a means of shrinking government and 'rolling back the state'. The benefits of this ideology and some of the concerns which have been expressed about it were considered in the previous chapter.

This chapter reviews the range of attitudes surrounding the policy implications of privatisation within the Criminal Justice System. In order to emphasise the different ideologies surrounding this policy, it specifically considers the privatisation of prisons. In the United States and Britain, this process has been stimulated both by ideological commitments and economic considerations. By tracing this development we consider the debate surrounding its implementation.

Although prison privatisation is not a new idea, the current wave of interest in the privatisation of corrections has been ongoing in the United States since about the mid-1970s and in the United Kingdom since the early 1980s This rekindling of interest grew as a response, primarily, to the issue of overcrowding and the escalating cost to the government of providing prisons for an increasing population of prisoners. In America, where the sociopolitical atmosphere has been one which has encouraged the notion of private enterprise, the free market and minimal state interference in the economy, this has produced a response which is both ideological and pragmatic in the sense that it helps to solve the penal crisis and at the same time reinforces the notion that the state should do less as a matter of principle. Faced with similar problems in the early 1980s, the British government sought to emulate this move towards the privatisation of correctional facilities. The Omega Justice Project outlined this possibility in 1988, emphasising that the crisis in overcrowding and cell sharing demanded reform of a radical nature, and pointed out that similar concerns in the United States, together with the cost to the American taxpayer, of imprisonment, had led to the adoption of new solutions to this problem. This included the use of independent firms to build, own and operate prisons and detention centres. It recommended that this could be the solution to similar problems faced by the prison system here, indicating that (p. 64):

> [i]t is surprising that the idea of independently built and managed prisons has not had a wider audience in Britain nor gained acceptance. Both security firms and hotel operations are commonplace in the private sector: it may be an oversimplification but a prison, borstal, or detention centre involves little more than a combination of these two talents. We suggest that the innovative methods of the private sector have a very important role to play in the provision of prisons in Britain, and that the government should take urgent steps to initiate private sector involvement.

This approach has brought about much debate in the political sphere and a number of concerns have been raised regarding its implementation. These are first, the conceptual and ethical issues involved in delegating the power to punish, and second, the legal, organisational and economic issues involved in the provision of these services. Before these issues are discussed, the nature and scope of correctional privatisation will briefly be addressed.

The Nature and Scope of Prison Privatisation

According to Shichor (1995, p. 1):

> [i]n the 1980's privatisation came primarily to mean two things: (1) any shift of activities from the state to the private sector; and (2) more specifically, any shift from public to private of the production of goods and services.

He indicates that in the United States this initially happened only in relation to services such as refuse collection and building maintenance, which he describes as 'hard services'. This was, however quickly extended to 'soft services' those termed as services performed 'for or on people', such as human services and public welfare. Included in this category are prisons, the privatisation of which can take many forms. According to Ryan and Ward (1989, pp. 3–4):

> it might mean that a private company builds, staffs and then runs a prison, receiving its clients, as it were, from the courts or indirectly from elsewhere in the penal system; or it could mean that a private company … builds a prison

and then rents it to the government of the day which then operates it with its own staff in the usual way ... it might also take the form of contracting out ... certain services, perhaps the provision of food or medicine.

Similarly, Shichor (1995) indicates that there are three major forms which the privatisation of prisons can take. These are (1) the private financing and construction of prisons, (2) private industry involvement in prisons and (3) the management and operation of a whole correctional facility by a private contractor, which he says is the most controversial area of privatisation.

As well as the sociopolitical ideologies associated with the move towards greater privatisation, other advantages of this move have been suggested. With the most recent crisis of overcrowding in prisons both in the United States and the United Kingdom it has been claimed that privatisation would increase available capacity because more prisons would be built more quickly. It has also been suggested that the introduction of competition would mean that a more innovative approach would be taken to correctional needs. Pease and Taylor (1989, p. 191) have outlined some of the possible advantages of privatisation, particularly in the commercial sense where they indicate that such ventures *need* results and that '[I]neffective penal sanctions ought to die. New options and improvements ought constantly to be sought'.

Chapter 1 outlined that the issue of privatisation in more general terms has had, and continues to receive, criticism. The suggestion of a greater move towards privatisation within the Criminal Justice System has systematically been the focus of a strong wave of specific criticism. This criticism has been associated most particularly in Britain with the political left, who have opposed the privatisation of the Criminal Justice System for a number of reasons, based broadly within the conceptual, ethical and organisational spheres. It is these issues which are now addressed.

Conceptual and Ethical Issues

Perhaps the most controversial of issues surrounding the implementation of privatisation in the Criminal Justice System is that which concerns the nature of the relationship between the state and the citizen and the functions which the state carries out (or *should* carry out) on behalf of its citizens.

Locke (1692) considered that through the notion of the social contract, the state was vested, by its citizens, with the power to maintain social order for the good of all. Therefore, the state had the power to punish if legal rules were violated because this was for the greater protection of all other citizens. Maguire (1985, p. 1) cites Disraeli as having said 'I repeat ... that all power is a trust – that we are accountable for its exercise – that, from the people, and for the people, all springs, and all must exist'.

Maguire (1985, p. 1) comments on this by saying that:

> Disraeli's fine rhetoric makes the concept and practice of accountability sound disarmingly simple. Power is seen as a trust held on behalf of 'the people', who must be satisfied by full and regular accounts ... that it is being exercised in a proper manner. But even the most cursory glance at the operation of contemporary state bureaucracies exposes the enormity of the gap between ideal and reality.

For some of the opponents of privatisation, this is the crux of the matter. It is contended that the power to punish is essentially vested in the state by the people and that it is only, and *should only* be administered by the state in its role of protecting society. Alternatively, it has been suggested that, despite this idea of the social contract, the ultimate political power still lies with the people who delegate it to those who govern. If this is not carried out properly, according to classical-liberal thinking, that power may be taken away from the state. Therefore, it is argued that the power to punish does not essentially lie solely with the state, but with all citizens who merely delegate that power to the state to act on their behalf. In this way, it is possible for right-wing proponents of correctional privatisation to argue that there is essentially no reason why the state should not delegate the power to punish back to its citizens. This is seen by some as a good way to shrink government which, according to Logan (1990) is increasingly usurping individual freedom. Therefore it is felt that there is a need to scale down state intervention in many areas including that of punishment. This is what is known as the 'libertarian' view of government of which the core ideas, according to Logan (1990, p. 239) are as follows:

1   individual rights are natural, inalienable and supreme;

2   the most fundamental of these are the rights to life, liberty and property;

3   no individual or group may rightfully initiate the use or threat of coercive force against anyone else;

4   within certain limits, individuals have the right to respond with force to the initiation or threat of force by others;

5 the state has no rights or legitimate powers not originally held by individuals, and therefore no unique claims to the legitimate use of force;

6 the proper function of government (if any) is to enforce and protect individual rights under the rule of law (reproduced from Shichor, 1995, p. 49).

The classical libertarian view illustrates that the power to punish belongs to the individual who may transfer this right legitimately to others. This is in direct conflict with the notion held by many opponents of the privatisation of the Criminal Justice System who argue that the state has the sole right to use legal coercive power and that if the machinery of justice is lain open to abuse this could, according to Matthews (1989, p. 1) '... undermine normative structures'.

These distinctions are at the heart of the debate about whether the administration of punishment, in whatever form, can be delegated successfully and equitably to the private sector. There are also questions regarding the propriety of providing such a service on a profit-making basis. DiIulio (1990, p. 73) contends that:

> on legitimate and moral grounds, the authority to govern those behind bars, to deprive citizens of their liberty, to coerce (and even kill) them, must remain in the hands of government authorities.

However, in contrast to this is the argument that in private correctional institutions, the management and personnel are still receiving their legal authority from the state and this creates an essential distinction between the power to impose punishment and the power to administer it, which can be seen as being two entirely separate functions.

Whatever stance is taken regarding this issue, it is clear that now the delegation of this sort of legitimate power *is* taking place both in the United States and the United Kingdom, the crucial point is to ensure that propriety and legal values, as well as control and accountability over those who are providing private services are maintained. According to Pease and Taylor (1989, p. 182):

> the critical question is not so much whether [private] prisons are run for profit but whether acceptable, relevant standards are applied to the provision and administration of facilities.

They also contend that after all, the idea of privatisation within the Criminal Justice System is not new. For example, Legal Aid is more like BUPA than the NHS, with private operators being reimbursed for services. Securicor run the Heathrow Airport detention facilities and certain services within the Criminal Justice System (such as food purchases) have always been largely contracted out. They conclude that '... the application of agreed standards, not a particular form of ownership, is the road to penological propriety'.

In contrast to this, DiIulio (1990) whilst accepting that private prisons could probably do everything that state-owned prisons do, is of the opinion that they should not do it as a matter of principle. His contention is that all administration and services for prisoners ought to be provided by the state. Contracting out prison services is seen as the 'thin end of the wedge' which could increase the likelihood of every part of the Criminal Justice System being privatised. If this were the case, would the police, Judges and juries be next? The implication here is that the move to greater privatisation could culminate in an 'all or nothing' scenario in which we must ultimately accept either total privatisation of all government authority and thus the complete dismantling of the state, or simply not have it at all.

In terms of the theoretical and conceptual issues surrounding privatisation and the Criminal Justice System, there are two conflicting views. Proponents expounding the libertarian view of the benefits of shrinking government and of the free market contend that privatising the delivery of punishment is nothing out of the ordinary and simply the next logical step in the progression of privatisation. Many accept that there are organisational problems connected with the delivery of private punishment but that these problems are entirely separate from the ideology itself and are not a bar to its successful implementation. Opponents maintain that the delivery of punishment is a role for the state alone and that in a complex society where the state has so many functions to perform, the ideology of a minimal state is not realistic. It is probably true that both sides agree that the delivery of punishment needs to be reviewed and should be more efficient, but there is an essential conflict of interests about the way in which this should be achieved.

In spite of this, the last 20 years has seen a dramatic rise in the interest and implementation of private prisons in the United States and Britain, a move which has been widely debated. The implementation of this policy and the debates surrounding it in both jurisdictions will now be addressed.

Prison Privatisation in the United States

Milton Friedman (1980, p. 1) describes the history of the United States as:

> an economic miracle and a political miracle that was made possible by the translation into practice of two sets of ideas – both, by a curious coincidence, formulated in documents published in the same year, 1776.

The ideas to which he refers are first, those embodied in Adam Smith's *The Wealth of Nations* and second, those embodied in Thomas Jefferson's Declaration of Independence. From these two documents came the essential ideas, as we saw in the previous chapter, of American economic and political freedom. It was also illustrated that from these ideologies came a resurgence of privatisation in the United States, from the 1970s onwards, as a measure aimed at curbing state and local expenditure, as well as fulfilling the political ideologies of what has been called the 'New Right'. Ryan and Ward (1989, p. 1) admit that in this political climate '[T]he recent suggestion that the delivery of punishment should be privatised ought not to surprise us'.

They describe President Reagan's Reform 88 Initiative as being designed specifically to involve the private sector more directly in what had previously only been public services, in an effort to curb expenditure at both federal and state levels. These efforts made privatisation an important political agenda from which it seemed no public utility was spared.

The ideology behind privatisation is often said to be that it offers a quick, cost-effective solution to many of the problems which face Western countries such as America and Britain. At this time, the penal system in both countries was under severe strain. In the United States, even medical or sanitary public services to prisons could not be guaranteed and overcrowding was getting worse. The only way to relieve this situation was to build more prisons, but how, at a time of limited financial resources, and without extra cost to the American taxpayer could this be achieved? The solution was to privatise the delivery of punishment. Doing this not only satisfied the political ideologies of the 'New Right' but also provided an economically feasible way of providing more prisons without incurring any further cost to the taxpayer or the government.

From the early 1980s, profit-making companies began to operate prisons in America. This, as indicated previously has taken three forms:

1 the private financing and construction of prisons. This allows for quicker

building of new prisons, the funds for which can be more easily secured through private financing than through public channels;

2   private industry involvement in prisons. Although this is not a new concept, there has been renewed interest in this idea since many proponents of privatisation support the inmates' need to learn skills, whilst in prison, that will be useful upon release;

3   management and operation of prisons by a private company.

Although this is not all that common, with the exception in America of juvenile corrective centres, it has been, and continues to be the most controversial.

All these methods have been used to implement the policy of prison privatisation in America. However, moves to deregulate and denationalise have not been without problems. The implementation of privatisation, both in terms of theory and practice has been one of great controversy, commented on by numerous writers. Camp and Camp (1985) studied contracted out services and the extent of the involvement of private companies in American correctional institutions. Their national study involved a survey mailed to 54 jurisdictions, with 52 agencies responding. At the time of their study, no secure adult facilities were privately operated, therefore their findings related only to services or programmes provided by the private sector. The study illustrated that there were both benefits and liabilities resulting from private sector involvement, their overview of this illustrating that:

> [g]enerally speaking, private sector services were considered more cost-effective than the same agency-provided ones. The most common problem was monitoring the performance of providers, closely followed by poor quality of service.. Administrators were most fond of medical service contracts because the provider can give better professional service and get better staff (1985, p. 15).

Elvin (1985) similarly provides some cautionary comments on the issue of private sector management of American jails, a move which has been attributed to a number of factors. Elvin suggests that these were the high cost of current prison operation in the United States, a huge prison population, public demand for stiffer sentences and pressure to improve existing prison conditions. Although there was a history of contractual arrangements between corrections agencies and private agencies, Elvin (1985, p. 49) suggests that 'private sector management and operation has gone largely untested'.

Elvin (1985, p. 51) indicates that the problems outlined stimulated an interest in the private sector management of prisons which in turn led to lively debate. Primarily she stresses concern over the ethical implications of such a move saying that:

> [t]his issue concerns us very deeply, since the delegation of the police power of the state to a private company is serious and troubling. We see the potential for serious abuse in the delegation of the control and custody of prisoners.

Concern is also expressed (1985, pp. 49–50) over the potential for lobbying for more prisoners by those involved in private provision: 'will entrepreneurs mobilize even further the already strong public and legislative support behind incarceration?'

In conclusion Elvin stresses that more attention should be paid to prisons in general to safeguard the correct implementation of society's rules and the rights of prisoners.

A further example is that of Travis et al. (1985, p. 11) who also make a plea for caution with regard to the growth and use of private prisons. They attribute this growth to a lack of faith in government provision as well as the growing demand of the early 1980s and cite the Camps' (1985) study as evidence that this is not a new phenomenon:

> [t]o be sure, there is ample evidence that certain government services can be provided in a more effective fashion by private companies. A survey conducted by the Camps (1984) revealed that some 52 agencies (both adult and juvenile) reported some 3,215 contracts with the private sector.

They establish that the involvement of the private sector in the prison industry is a long one, early prisons being operated by individuals who did this for profit. However, they also reveal that the change to a state-run system of prisons was an attempt to alleviate the abuses of this early system in which many prisoners were exploited. The current return of interest in private sector involvement in prisons is new however, from the point of view that it is not just the provision of goods and services which was proposed, but the establishment of contract facilities, to be built and run by the private sector, on a profit making basis. It is this that Travis et al. discuss. Outlining some of the benefits anticipated by the advocates of this system Travis et al. (1985, p. 13) suggest that:

> [t]he promise of private involvement in correctional services is the promise of

the free market. Several companies in competition with each other for the correctional market and guided by the profit motive should be able to provide better, cheaper correctional services than can the current governmental monopoly.

They also cite Don Hutto, Director of the Corrections Corporation of America who has claimed that one of the benefits of prison privatisation is that:

> [t]he private corporation can 'cut red tape' ... [and] cut through the layers of protection established in government and build new facilities in a shorter time with greater access to private capital. Private corporations are able to build without resorting to a public referendum by attracting private investors eager for tax breaks which lease-purchase or service contracts typically offer.

Hutto has also suggested that such contracts are advantageous to governments because they force a situation whereby the government must produce a contract clearly stating the relationship between itself and the contractor and the services to be provided.

Having outlined some of the benefits of such a system, Travis et al. also discuss the problems of private involvement in the areas of legality, cost and accountability. In terms of legality, they suggest that it is of prime importance that contracts entered into between the government and a private company must contain guidelines regarding the use of coercive power and how these powers (usually seen as being solely within the exercise of the state) might be delegated. Second they suggest (p. 14) that 'it is by no means certain that a contract institution would be more cost-effective than its government counterpart' and that whilst they accept that the profit motive *might* provoke the incentive for efficiency in theory, it does not necessarily mean that this would be realised in practice.

Finally they address the issue of accountability. Although they admit that it is possible to introduce more effective private business practices into the public sector, this does not mean that all private companies are totally efficient and accountable and all public sector ones are incompetent. The aim should be to introduce the public sector to a more sound, businesslike approach and methods which would accordingly benefit the industry. If then, the government is to relinquish the management of facilities to a private operator, they must still be accountable for the delivery of these services and this requirement must be specified in any contract.

In conclusion, Travis et al. (1985, p. 15) remain unconvinced about private sector involvement in prisons and suggest that:

given that public jails and prisons were developed as a response to the inadequacies of private institutions, there is a danger that returning to past practices will lead to more problems than it will resolve. Rather than return to the solutions of the past, we would urge that we look to solutions for the future.

This illustrates that the move towards greater involvement of the private sector in the management of correctional facilities in the United States has provoked strong reactions, in spite of the American culture of the free market and private sector involvement in many other areas of American life. The emergence of this idea and its implementation in the United Kingdom is now considered.

Prison Privatisation in the United Kingdom

Although the idea of privatisation in the United Kingdom is certainly not new, for Britain in the postwar period, it had become the norm for the state to be seen as the natural provider of services like health, education and the Criminal Justice System. We have seen that the current trend in deregulation and denationalisation was initially advocated by Margaret Thatcher's government which began, in the early 1980's, to withdraw the state from the production of many goods and services. This was carried out in order to achieve both the ideological, political and economic goals of the Conservatives who, according to Veljanovski (1988, p. 2) believe that it:

> enhances individual freedoms, encourages and improves efficiency, makes industry more responsive to the demand of the customer, decreases the public debt and weakens the power of the trade unions by forcing management to face the realities of the market place.

The response to this policy has been illustrated to have been mixed. However, proposals to include parts of the Criminal Justice System within this framework have probably elicited the most criticism on the basis of the moral and ethical issues involved. These were addressed earlier in this chapter.

The motivation behind the idea of privatising (in some form) British prisons was probably initially voiced by the Adam Smith Institute. Young (1988, p. 2) argued that:

> British prisons share the same characteristics as other public sector institutions that are immune from competition: inadequate supply, low quality and high

cost. Any reform proposals must address this issue of monopoly provision as the source of much of the difficulty besetting the prison service today, and should not confine its analysis only to the specific issues of crime and punishment techniques. That is why the move towards private prisons in America holds out so much hope for Britain. By introducing an element of competition into the British prison business, one should be able to increase supply, improve quality and reduce cost.

Like the American prison system, the British prison system was also in need of review and reform. Overcrowding, violence, rooftop sieges and industrial disputes were fairly common. Like America, prison overcrowding was a problem because government policy put spending on health and education as a higher priority. It was these problems which, in part, led the government to look at the United States experience of privately managed prisons as a possible model for similar introduction in Britain. Young (1988, p. 38) reported on a study of the private prison experience in the United States and commented that:

> [p]erhaps the most surprising facts revealed by the report are the greatly improved conditions for prisoners in all the United States private jails. These improved conditions have been hailed by the prisoners themselves and by disinterested observers such as local media and clergy. That costs can be cut is not very surprising, given the general record of privatisation, but that private firms can both cut costs and improve standards is certainly worth noting. Perhaps the most compelling argument for prison privatisation is therefore the humanitarian one.

Glowing reports of the American experience led the British government in the 1980s seriously to consider the introduction of private prisons in the United Kingdom. Now, not only did it have its ideological commitments and the current economic prison crisis as reasons for moving towards this, but it was able also to cite the success of the American prison privatisation experience in defence of this policy.

Ryan and Ward (1989, p. 45) attribute much of the government's interest in prison privatisation to the work of the Adam Smith Institute. In Britain, the ASI is a registered charity, but was originally founded in America in 1978. It was responsible, in 1984, for the Omega Report on Justice Policy, which outlined privatisation as a possible means of solving the prison crisis by 'concentrating resources on capital investment rather than increased labour costs'.

Ryan and Ward (1989) suggest that this was not taken very seriously at the time, but subsequently, as a result of Peter Young's work in America,[1] *The*

Prison Cell was published by ASI in 1987. This advocated the benefits of the privatisation of prisons based on the United States experience and was also endorsed by a Conservative Study Group on Crime (1986).

Culmination of the interest in the prison crisis and suggestions for its resolution prompted the Home Affairs Select Committee, in 1987, to examine the state and use of prisons. In fact finding for their third report they travelled to the United States specifically to view a number of prisons, some of which were run by the Corrections Corporation of America (CCA). From this time a more marked interest in the privatisation of prisons issue began to grow and was subsequently discussed in the Committee's fourth report, entitled *Contract Provision of Prisons*. This report suggested that the private provision of penal establishments would:

1 relieve the taxpayer of the immediate burden of having to pay for their initial capital cost;

2 dramatically accelerate [prison] building;

3 produce greatly enhanced architectural efficiency and excellence (reproduced from Ryan and Ward, 1989, p. 53.)

The problem of overcrowding was one which was particularly highlighted. This was attributed to large numbers of remand prisoners. As a result the private provision of remand prisons became a particular point of focus for the government culminating in the spring of 1988 in the Home Office publication 'Private Sector Involvement in the Remand System'. Subsequently tenders were invited by the government, for build-only contracts for open prisons and remand centres and a little later the Home Secretary invited management consultants Deloitte Haskins and Sells to report on the practicality of private sector involvement in the remand system. The Deloitte Consultancy Report was supervised by the Home Office Remand Unit and representatives of the Home Office and Lord Chancellor's Department. They concluded that the scheme for private sector involvement was feasible and importantly, that effective monitoring could be achieved by Board of Visitors and HM Inspectorate of Prisons, also that a move in this direction would cut costs, benefit prisoners and help to relieve pressure on prison officers and the police.

The consultancy report therefore echoed the views of the Select Committee on Home Affairs, but this was merely the start of a much wider debate regarding this policy and its implementation, in which emotions ran very high.

Some examples of this can be found in the report of the ISTD (Institute for the Study and Treatment of Delinquency) conference 'Punishment for Profit' which took place in 1989 and more recently in the Hansard Report of the parliamentary debate which took place on 3 February 1993. The former will be discussed first.

As one of the opponents, Roger Matthews considered that, aside from the conceptual and ethical problems associated with providing private punishment, the question of whether prison privatisation would cut the cost of the criminal justice system was worth addressing since he agreed that the amount of public money involved in it had reached what he called 'astronomic proportions'. However, he went on to say that there were a number of problems in determining whether this would be a cost-cutting exercise. The first was that it would be difficult to make a comparison between public and private sector provision because there is a lack of financial information available to make this comparison feasible. Second, he proposed that whilst a move in this direction may mean some savings, it would also mean greater administrative provision, since it was not being suggested that state power should be relinquished in the realm of criminal justice. Therefore, to hold private agencies accountable in this field and to monitor them effectively would naturally entail considerable cost. He also expressed doubts about the efficacy of providing yet more prisons, citing Douglas Hurd as having admitted that putting criminals in prison only served to make them more skilful offenders when they were released. In the light of this, Matthews raised the issue of the government Green Paper which had [then] recently proposed two new prisons and questioned the need for them on the basis of a cost-cutting exercise. He suggested (1989, p. 29) that:

> [a] more realistic approach would extend the use of the fine and link it to the offender's ability to pay ... would endeavour to make legal services accessible and affordable for all ... [and] encourage the private sector to show their appreciation of the services provided on their behalf by the criminal justice system and invite them – particularly when they err – to make substantial contributions to the costs of providing this service. Having effected some or all of these changes we might begin to develop a more cost-effective criminal justice system.

At the same conference other cautious comments on the subject were made by Stephen Shaw, Director of the Prison Reform Trust. His view was that whilst he accepted that some privatisation of the penal system was inevitable, he was not prepared to assume that the battle was lost. From an ethical point of view he did not feel that, just because the Americans were adjudged by the government to have made a success of it, this meant it was alright for Britain to do it. Farrell (1989, p. 52) quotes him thus:

[w]e do not have to incorporate American values – particularly those from the southern states where the exploitation of prisoners has been greatest historically. In the United States they sell blood. In this country, even the Prime Minister was appalled by the 'kidney vendor' schemes run by private hospitals.

Other main concerns he expressed were that this move would mean intolerable variations in prison standards. He also showed concern over standards being consistently upheld, saying that:

[i]f we can guarantee openness and enforce the standards, then private prisons could provide an opportunity for new protections for prisoners and, ultimately, for the establishment of minimum standards throughout the system – public and private alike.

However, he remained fairly unconvinced, calling the Deloitte Report 'feeble' and 'full of unsubstantiated comments'. He also used Harmondsworth Immigration Detention Centre (privately managed for 20 years) as an example of private sector involvement and said that Judge Tumim thought it 'poor value for money' and was 'not convinced of its efficiency'. Besides that, it was not making a profit.

In spite of being highly critical of the Deloitte Report, Shaw acknowledged to some extent its recommendations regarding contracts, standards and evaluation criteria, but concluded that (Farrell (1989, p. 51):

[i]t is not my view that the state must enjoy a monopoly of everything in the criminal justice system ... I believe that there may be a very creative role in such areas as prison industries, catering, recreation, counselling and so on ... In contrast, the sub-contracting of whole institutions raises many dangers. Not least it raises the spectre of a lobby with a vested interest in the higher prison population.

In response to this Sir Edward Gardner QC (1989, pp. 13–4) a proponent of privatisation, and (at the time of the reports mentioned above) Chairman of the Select Committee on Home Affairs, expressed the opinion that '[t]he heart of the problem ... is overcrowding ... the root cause [of which] is the presence among the prison population of remand prisoners'.

This, he said was the reason why the Select Committee had looked at private sector involvement in the American penal system and why Deloitte, Haskins and Sells were asked by the government to look at the feasibility of introducing it to Britain. Taking exception to what Stephen Shaw expressed about the report he commented (1989, p. 16):

> [n]ow, of course, when you don't like something and the document before you says something which you find disagreeable, one way of dealing with this is to rubbish it and that, if you will allow me to say so, is just what Stephen Shaw tries to do with great skill in his paper. I only bring the technique to your attention in order that you will not be deceived by it, for in fact, Deloitte, Haskins and Sells, in whose commercial or any other interest I have no part whatsoever, have an outstanding reputation so good that the Government chose them to carry out this particular job.

In relation to the issue of overcrowding, his view was that the separate, possibly private provision of remand prisons was the only feasible solution to this problem and that he was convinced by the Deloitte Report which had recommended that the idea was feasible and that effective safeguards and monitoring could be achieved and that it would reduce costs and relieve unnecessary pressure on prison officers. With regard to the question of whether punishment for profit was ethical he said this question was (1989, p. 16):

> irrelevant because what I have been putting before you and what was put before the government by the Select Committee on Home Affairs had nothing to do with punishment as such. The people who would control the size of population in a remand centre would have nothing to do with the private sector ... [this] would be entirely within the jurisdiction of the courts.

At the conference, Farrell (1989, p. 11) cites other supporters of privatisation including Robert Fulton, Head of the Home Office Remands Unit and Don Hutto, Director of the Corrections Corporation of America. Fulton raised the issue that these ideas were indeed nothing new and that in fact it was Jeremy Bentham who had first suggested contract prisons in about 1810, for the sole reason that they would then be open to scrutiny.

> Many of the arguments and ideas which he advanced strangely parallel the debate which is taking place today. In his proposals, the contractor's self-interest and that of the prisoners would be brought together in a system of incentives and penalties which rewarded the contractor for looking after the prisoners properly and penalised him if he did not. In these circumstances, the profit motive was seen as a force for good.

Similarly, Hutto dismissed the ethical arguments against this sort of provision (1989, p. 23):

> [t]he proposition that profiting from people's misery is immoral conveniently ignores the fact that profit centres emerge around all human endeavours, and criminal justice has been no exception.

His view was that the fostering of competition would bring improvement, that agencies would be able to work together, with the government then in a position to oversee the delivery and quality of the service being provided. He also dismissed the suggestion that the government would not be able to do this in the following way:

> [t]o suggest that government is capable of safeguarding the rights of prisoners by monitoring facilities which government itself operates but is incapable of safeguarding the rights of prisoners when monitoring privately managed ones is inconsistent and without foundation.

The expression of these views illustrates that emotions ran high initially. The following description of the Hansard Report of the Draft Criminal Justice Act 1991 (Contracted Out Prisons) (No. 2) Order 1992, debated on 3 February 1993 demonstrates that this was also the case recently.

At the time of this debate, two private prisons had already been opened. These were The Wolds Remand Prison and Blakenhurst which holds both remand and sentenced prisoners. The debate focused on the above order which was designed to allow the management of existing prisons to be contracted out to private operators and sparked a heated debate in the House which was published in Hansard (1993) and from which all the following quotations are derived.

The (then) Home Secretary, Kenneth Clarke began the debate by outlining the benefits of the new system, including the establishment of good practices and the introduction of valuable new ideas.

> The performance of prisons will be closely and continually monitored to ensure compliance with the high standards that we have set out in the agreement with the contractor. In debating the contracting out of prisons, we should look at the positive programme that we have put in place by setting out the specifications that are in line with the Woolf Report (1993, p. 420).

The Home Secretary then went on to say that the government was well on the way to a significant amount of this sort of private sector involvement and that it felt this was good because it would achieve better conditions for prisoners whilst at the same time benefiting the taxpayer. He stressed the element of competition which he said would help to bring about better standards which were in line with the recommendations of Lord Justice Woolf and Judge Tumim.

In response to this Tony Blair agreed that there should be reform of the prison system, but did not agree that it should be done in this way. He felt that privatisation was a diversion from the actual issue and that in principle the idea was fundamentally flawed and 'pursued for reasons which have nothing to do with efficiency or prison reform but are simply an obsession with the idea of privatisation itself' (1993, p. 426).

His opinion was that privatisation of the prison service would create confusion resulting from a multiplicity of contracts with different contractors and that any benefits described from existing prisons like The Wolds or Blakenhurst were not the outcome of privatisation at all.

> That is the sham at the heart of it. They are the outcome of the government specifying the regime at the prison. It has nothing to do with the private sector or the public sector and everything to do with the government being prepared to implement the very specifications that we have been asking for the whole of the prison service (1993, p. 428).

In a similar context the MP Gerald Bermingham raised the issue of profit, asking what advantage it was to make a profit from imprisoning someone and why a private individual should be able to offer something that the state could not. This point was taken up by Tony Blair who agreed that it was essentially wrong for people to be imprisoned by other than the state. He felt that the issue of accountability was in question and that such companies would not be accountable to the government, as the Home Secretary had said, but to their shareholders. He was of the opinion that:

> to allow a private security company, whose main motivation must be commercial, the coercive powers of detention, punishment, physical restraint and influence on decisions about parole – powers of a real and harsh nature – is wrong in principle and should not be countenanced by the House.

In contrast to this, the MP Sir John Wheeler proposed that the use of the term 'privatisation' in this context was not necessarily appropriate since the debate concerned market testing and the use of accountable management contracts. In this respect he could:

see no reason why an accountable contract should not lead to a better standard of service for the public interest, with better conditions for prison inmates and an improvement in the quality of training and facilities. I also believe that it is essential to allow people who work in the prison system the variety of other experiences. Such ideas are commonplace in the United States (1993, p. 430).

This point was taken up by the Home Secretary who maintained that legal authority in such circumstances was ultimately derived from the House and this would be the case even in private prisons who would have a controller based there as a Crown servant to ensure that this happened. The MP Robert Maclennan was amongst others who were not swayed by this statement, saying that:

> [i]t is open to a private citizen to use force to restrain a member of the public who is committing a crime. The Home Secretary need not teach his grandmother tricks on such a matter. The question whether it is appropriate to place prison guards in a position where they have to use force as a matter of course, day in, day out, without the advantage of professional training … is at least debatable. Many people doubt it is a suitable policy (1993, p. 434).

In response to this Sir Ivan Lawrence voiced his surprise at the views of the opposition whom he took as wishing to see more humane prison conditions. This, he said was an opportunity to achieve better conditions which the Labour party (who in the light of a 15 per cent rise in prison population cut capital spending on prisons by 20 per cent from 1974 to 1979) was unable to achieve themselves.

At this point, referring back to the comments of Sir John Wheeler, the MP Barbara Roche expressed her concern over the comparisons that were being drawn between Britain and the United States, whose interest in the privatisation of prisons she termed 'obnoxious' because 'companies such as Kentucky Fried Chicken [had] been involved in tenders and indeed, the running of some prisons. Is that not a bizarre and atrocious way to run the system?'[2]

She also criticised the Wolds for being an expense to the taxpayer, although the exact figures were not known because the government, she said, would not reveal them. She also accused the government of planning to hand out the contracts for the management of such prisons to the Secretary of State's friends.

At this point, having discussed the motion for 90 minutes, this rather emotionally charged debate ended with a vote in favour of the order. This does, however, give some indication of how strong feelings were in parliament, in relation to these moves.

Given that these issues were debated with such vigour, it is interesting briefly to mention reports of how successfully prison privatisation has been implemented by reference to reports which have since been made regarding both The Wolds and Blakenhurst.

Blakenhurst was inspected by HM Chief Inspector of Prisons Judge Tumim in May 1994, one year after it had opened. Judge Tumim acknowledged that this was a relatively short time for the prison to become properly established and was reported in Prison Report (1995, p. 13) as saying that:

> after a shaky start the prison was beginning to stabilise ... the most impressive feature [being] the quality, enthusiasm and potential of staff: the most disappointing feature was the comparative shortage of innovation.

In his report, published in February 1995, Judge Tumim noted some positive and negative aspects to Blakenhurst. On the positive side some of the following comments were made:

- the quality, enthusiasm and motivation of prison officers was impressive and the number of incidents few, owing to their good dispositions and relations with the inmates;

- the building was clean and well maintained and staff working conditions were good;

- physical security was good, the monitoring of the treatment of prisoners was good and excessive use of control and restraint techniques had been cut back;

- the education service was outstanding;

- three-quarters of the population enjoyed an out of cell regime of 13–14 hours a day;

- one of the most impressive aspects of the prison was the reception process; the computerised system recording every prisoner's photograph and custodial details were impressive. Each new reception was issued with an electronic wristband and the system had great potential.

On the negative side, Judge Tumim made some of the following comments:

- an attempt to merge United States and United Kingdom cultures had resulted in a lack of clarity between roles. The top management structure was complex and lacked clarity. The director had little scope for decision making. There was little evidence of clear policy planning within a strategic framework;

- no formal policy to combat bullying;

- senior managers worked long hours and after 12 months were feeling the effects of complying with the contract;

- prisoners had a range of concerns including limited recreational facilities; instances of being produced at court although they were not required to be there; vulnerable prisoners were not given a copy of the rules and relatives and friends were kept waiting a long time before visits got under way;

- quality of throughcare for prisoners was poor;

- nine major assaults on other prisoners and 54 technical assaults on staff had occurred (reproduced from Prison Report, 1995, pp. 13–4.)

In the same issue, Prison Report commented that Blakenhurst was given eight months to respond to Judge Tumim's report. In doing so, it redefined the responsibilities of middle managers and appointed an experienced middle manager to strengthen the team. It also developed a comprehensive programme to help prisoners confront their offending behaviour as well as setting up a sex-offender assessment course and constructing an anti-bullying strategy. It had also given prisoners unrestricted access to a direct telephone line to the Samaritans.

Blakenhurst has received less public and media scrutiny than the Wolds Remand Prison, which was the first to be contracted out, the operation of which was won by Group 4 Securities.

The Wolds opened in April 1992 and is situated 12 miles west of Hull. Reports of the prison since it opened have been on the whole favourable, despite great initial resistance. Bean (1992, p. 1610) describes the Wolds as very different from any state-run establishment, having a low-key, relaxed atmosphere and a noticeable absence of shouting, inmates and staff being summoned as needed by a PA system. One prisoner is described as saying:

> I didn't know what to expect when I knew I was coming here. But when I arrived I couldn't believe it. You go to Hull or Leeds and they treat you like cattle, but I walked in this place and they gave me a cup of tea and switched the telly on.

The Wolds has a director, not a governor and the management team was recruited from state prisons. Other staff were recruited either from state prisons, or locally, many being completely new to prison work and having undergone a period of training. The prison itself is built on two storeys around a recreational area on the ground floor and prisoners remain outside their cells for at least 14 hours a day. Complaints from prisoners are few and Bean comments that (1992, p. 1610):

> [t]he inmates may prefer it to any state-run prison but they are all very temporary residents. Soon they will go to court, most to receive a prison sentence. The stark contrast between the modern, comfortable surroundings they have left and the Victorian fortresses of Armley or Hull will do nothing to improve an already volatile prison situation.

For this reason it is reported that many prisoners try to serve the majority of their sentence at the Wolds by spinning out court dates. In spite of such reports, opponents still say that prisons should not be privatised and that profiting from other people's misery is wrong. But as Bean (1992, p. 1610) comments 'the prisoners of the Wolds would say that they are suffering far less misery there than in any state-run remand prison'.

In 1992 the Home Office Research and Planning Unit (now the Research and Statistics Directorate) commissioned a study of the Wolds Remand Prison to evaluate key aspects of the design and operation of the regime there and to compare these with concurrent developments in new public sector prisons. The study was conducted by Keith Bottomley, Adrian James and Emma Clare (University of Hull) and Alison Liebling (Cambridge Institute of Criminology) with the main fieldwork taking place between November 1992 and October 1993 with follow-up visits until March 1994. Although the full report was not available to me at the time, a summary of the research findings was and this outlines the key points of the findings in the following way:

* Wolds management and Group 4 succeeded in running this new prison for its first two years with relatively few major incidents, none of which involved loss of control of the prison;

- nearly 80 per cent of prisoners at Wolds regarded it as better than other prisons which they had experienced. Although a small minority felt unprotected and vulnerable, the majority supported the contracting-out of more prisons insofar as this would lead to improved conditions for prisoners;

- however, comparable achievements were to be found in some public sector local prisons. There was therefore no evidence that Wold's achievements were necessarily related to its contracted-out status;

- both staff and prisoners identified the quality of staff-prisoner relationships as being one of the most important aspects of Wolds, but staff saw the price paid as high in terms of long shifts and high levels of isolation. The majority of prisoners spoke highly of the staff working at Wolds;

- although staffing levels did not lead directly to any serious compromises in the security of the prison, there were situations in which higher levels of staffing might have improved the maintenance of order and helped to reduce staff concerns about their potential vulnerability;

- there are a few simple conclusions which can be drawn about the advantages or disadvantages of the private sector compared with the public sector. There were more similarities in the tasks which all senior prison managers had to address than there were clear-cut differences in the way these tasks were tackled according to the 'private v. public' dimension (reproduced from Home Office, 1996).

The paper concludes by saying (1996, p. 4) that:

> [p]rivate sector prisons should remain under close professional and public scrutiny. The Controller's role remains a vital safeguard for public and political accountability and for ensuring the proper observation of prisoners' rights and interests, in particular the application of the disciplinary system.

Discussion

This chapter has addressed the moves towards the privatisation of prisons in America and Britain. Here, the policy has been consistent with the Conservative government's overall denationalisation programme, was lobbied for by the

New Right and the Adam Smith Institute and was given support by the Home Affairs Select Committee. It has also been consistently opposed by the political left, and, amongst others, the Howard League and the Prison Officer's Association

Lilly and Knepper (1992, p. 5) comment that this has been an international trend with Western practices of imprisonment creating a market for companies which specialise in the corrections business. They have suggested that this trend is one of 'correctional policy imperialism' and that:

> the relationship between the two nations is not based on the transfer of correctional policy so much as it is on the joint ownership of corporations that profit from marketing corrections products and services. Corrections Corporation of America, the most celebrated private prison corporation has well-known corporate roots. It is backed by the Massey-Burch Investment Group, owner of Kentucky Fried Chicken and the Hospital Corporation of America ... Other private firms are truly transnational. Group 4 International Corrections Services Inc received England's first contract for privately managing its new Wolds prison.

Whatever the relationship between the United Kingdom and the United States in the corrections market, the next stage in Britain's denationalisation policy has sought to include the privatisation of mental health care. This was touched on by the Home Secretary during the parliamentary debate on the contracting out of prisons where he commented (1993, p. 426) that:

> [w]e need to improve facilities and the problem of those who require psychiatric care in prisons has always been, and remains, serious ... I would like private sector prisons and operators to contract for their medical care from outside. That is one way of introducing a variety of approaches to the system so that we can raise the medical regimes inside prisons up to the standards we would like to see.

The next chapter outlines the development of private mental health care and its origins in the American experience.

Notes

1   Peter Young was the former head of research for the ASI and carried out more of their research into private prisons, having also worked at the American ASI office in Virginia.
2   The reference to Kentucky Fried Chicken is used because the Corrections Corporation of America (a well-known American private prison corporation) is backed by the Massey-Burch Investment Group who own, amongst other things, the Kentucky Fried Chicken chain (Home Office, 1993).

3 Private Mental Health Care

Private health care and more specifically private mental health care in the United Kingdom and abroad is not a new idea. Literature suggests that there have been moves towards this in countries as diverse as Canada, Australia, Hong Kong, New Zealand and Italy. However, in the United Kingdom, literature on the recently expanding market in private psychiatric provision is extremely limited and the impact of this move has not yet been fully explored.

In the United States, where health care is predominantly private, the implications of this sort of move have been monitored far more extensively. In relation to psychiatry, which Dorwat et al. (1988) say was not extensively privatised until the 1960s, there has been a renewed debate surrounding this issue and as such it provides an excellent point of comparison. It is relevant therefore to review the current American literature on this and to determine the prevalence of, attitudes to, success and potential problems of private mental health care in the United States in a way which will provide a feasible and useful backdrop for the United Kingdom.

In order to provide a background for this, the nature of current private medical care and private psychiatric care in the United Kingdom will first be discussed briefly.

Private Medical Care

Private medical or health care refers to the utilisation of health resources outside those provided by the National Health Service, the word 'private' being derived from the Latin *privatus* which means 'apart from the state.' This appears at first sight to be a good definition because it emphasises the essential distinction between the two. However, in doing so it obviously also ignores the fact that there can often be an overlap between the public and private sectors and differing realms of discourse existing in relation to them. Other definitions of private medical care may depend on who is giving them. For instance, the medical profession may well give a definition which stresses the professional input which is involved, whereas a patient might emphasise the notion of

41

'opting out of the NHS' or the idea of choosing to pay for treatment which might otherwise be available without charge. In both cases, these definitions are unsatisfactory because they ignore essential facts such as the possible interaction between the public and private sectors which can exist and which make it possible for specialists to work in both spheres and for patients to be treated in both sometimes irrespective of the element of charge. The public and private sectors cannot, therefore, be treated as entirely separate entities. A much better way to look at private medical care is in contractual terms, where doctors are no longer in a contractual relationship with the state and can therefore determine their own fees for their own services and where most often, the patient takes on the responsibility for paying that fee, usually through insurance (although in practice BUPA and others often have guideline fees above which they will not pay).

Turning now to the scope of private medical care, this also gives rise to a discussion of what has been voiced frequently as one of the major concerns in this area – that of the ownership of private health care facilities.

There are basically three main categories of ownership of private health care facilities of various types in the United Kingdom. These are: a) British profit-making firms; b) overseas profit-making firms; and c) charitable and religious organisations

The first category is financed and run commercially and although some forms are owned by private individuals or partnerships, given the costs involved and the need to guarantee returns sufficient to cover the costs of their development, large companies are often involved in their financing.

The second category of investment is by overseas companies. Most are American. These include companies such as American Medical International (A.M.I.) now called Partnerships in Care, who own, amongst others, Stockton Hall Psychiatric Hospital, York, which forms one site of this study. Such companies have not limited themselves to one speciality but have extended to cover a range of medical and surgical activities throughout the country and will obviously continue to do so if sufficient returns are likely.

The third category is the most long-standing one. Charitable and religious organisations date from before the inception of the NHS. More recently however, due to rising costs and the advancement of technology, they have often merged with other hospitals and now do not have such a significant role in the sphere of private health care. The one exception to this is the Nuffield Hospital chain which was founded in 1957 as a charity. Until 1984, Nuffield was the largest private hospital chain in the United Kingdom, but this position has since been taken over by Partnerships in Care (Home Office, 1991).

Private Psychiatric Provision in England and Wales

Until recently, all psychiatric inpatient treatment was provided by the public sector. Patients could be treated either in the psychiatric unit of a general hospital, in one of the Regional Secure Units, (in conditions of medium security) or, in the most serious of cases, in one of the maximum security Special Hospitals. The growth and current prevalence of the private sector in the speciality of medium secure facilities has arisen from a lack of beds within the public sector. This has, in part, been attributed to the process of closing many psychiatric facilities within the United Kingdom, and deinstitutionalising their former populations. The lack of provision of medium secure psychiatric beds is documented by a variety of sources, including most authoritatively the Reed Report (1992). Against this background, it is not surprising that there has been a dramatic increase in the number of secure psychiatric beds being provided by the private sector over recent years. Partnerships in Care plc (previously A.M.I. plc) now provides in excess of 300 secure private psychiatric beds. When one takes into account private sector care being provided by other independent operators, such as St Andrew's Hospital, Northampton, and compares it against the total of little more than 700 medium secure psychiatric beds provided by the National Health Service in England and Wales, (Coid, 1991) it is apparent that private health care organisations are providing a fairly significant proportion (30 per cent) of the total medium secure psychiatric accommodation available. With very few exceptions (Coid, 1993) the literature on the expanding market in private secure psychiatric care is extremely limited. The growth of private secure psychiatric provision is, however, an important development. Its examination is both appropriate and necessary.

Secure psychiatric care is relatively expensive, costing in excess of £200 a day. These charges are normally borne by the Health Authority from which the patient originates (and therefore most usually not from the patients themselves) so there must be the necessary impetus for the referring authority to fund a private bed. This sort of referral most often falls into one of four categories. First, a patient clearly requires admission, due to severe psychiatric disturbance, for which there is no bed available in his or her home district, a continuously pressing problem for health authorities with too few beds, as documented by Watson (1994). In such instances, the local authority may have little alternative but to fund a private bed. The second category of patient comprises individuals who, through long-term severe management problems, generally due to repetitive assaultive behaviour upon others, or repetitive self-injury have caused such severe difficulties in their local services, with the accompanying resource implications, that it is 'worth the while' of the parent authority to fund private care. The third category involves patients whose 'political sensitivity' necessitates the provision of a psychiatric bed. There is often a forensic history to such cases. Examples include patients for whom a bed is requested by the Court, or a serving prisoner, where a bed is requested by the Home Office, when, in the absence of a suitable placement in the home area, failure to provide alternative psychiatric provision through a funding in the private sector would be an embarrassment to the parent authority. Finally, there is the practice of referring to the independent sector patients who are deemed to require medium secure psychiatric care on a protracted basis. This reflects the absence of long-term medium secure provision within the National Health Service, where regional secure units are only prepared to accept patients who require their services for two years or less.

It is to be expected that private organisations will to some extent be motivated by the potential for profit that their services provide, and in this context, the current lack of adequate secure psychiatric care provides an attractive business opportunity. Whatever role the profit motive plays in the provision of such services, it is clear that the private sector is making a numerically important contribution to difficult or forensic patients who require secure care. The competitive aspects of market forces can be expected to ensure that referrals receive prompt attention and hopefully also encourage the provision of high quality clinical services. There may also, however, be areas of potential concern in this expanding market. Unlike private medicine, within the acute and surgical fields, where the 'customer' is the patient, in private secure psychiatric care, the 'customer' is the referring health authority which is paying for the service provided. Most patients admitted to private secure psychiatric care are detained under the terms of the Mental Health Act 1983 and are not there of their own volition. An increased emphasis has therefore to be placed on the purchasing authority to monitor the quality of the care provided, in order to guard against the quest for profit taking undue precedence at the expense of maintaining expected clinical standards. This may be difficult when the patient's home health authority is some distance away from the independent hospital providing service. Coid (1993) points out that patients placed in private psychiatric care are often transported considerable distances from their homes. Besides the unfortunate aspects of dislocating patients from their home areas – a concern documented by the Reed Committee – note has also to be made of the problems of private health care operators in offering psychiatric follow-up and continuation of care following discharge. At this point, the responsibility for the patient is generally handed back to clinicians within the patient's home area. There may also be financial pressures upon the private health care business which necessitate keeping unoccupied beds to a minimum. This might have the potential for tempting such organisations into accepting patients for whom their services are not appropriate. There is however corresponding pressure on public sector provision, which should not go unremarked. Presently, all regional psychiatric care is bought in advance by that region's purchasing authority. Contracts are agreed between the purchasing authority and public sector providers for the psychiatric care that district's patients are likely to need during the year. Therefore if public sector providers do not give a good service, it is likely that the purchasing authority will not renew its contract with them the following year. So, there is pressure on each side.

Having made these cautionary notes, the limited literature on private secure psychiatric care speaks positively of the quality of the care being provided. To date, however, there are no published studies comparing care and programmes available in the private and National Health Service sectors and as such, there is a need for more information regarding how the independent sector is operating in this field and meeting the national need for medium secure psychiatric provision. The later chapters of this study will seek to redress the balance by addressing these issues and providing evidence of empirical study comparing programmes available in the private and public sectors in the United Kingdom, in the area of medium security. First, what follows is a literature review of similar provision in the USA which will provide an interesting backdrop for this work.

Private Psychiatric Provision in the USA

Although the American health care system is dominated by the private sector, one exception to this has been mental health care. Approximately 90 per cent was provided by public facilities until the 1960s when a significant and widely remarked move towards the privatisation of psychiatric care started to take place. By the mid 1980s it was reported (O'Connor, 1984) that approximately 60 per cent of the psychiatric proprietary hospitals in the United States were investor-owned.

In his 1978 article, Gibson outlines the historical background to this. He describes American private psychiatric hospitals as having always been a major force in psychiatry and one which had consistently adopted a moral, humane and forward-thinking approach with regard to the mentally ill. He explains the greater interest in and emphasis on private psychiatric care as being the result of an increase in 'psychiatric patient care episodes' (1978, p. 17) which in turn led to a growth in new investor-owned hospitals, which were responding to a gap in the market. Gibson points out that by 1975, of all the private psychiatric hospitals in America, two-thirds were owned by corporations, individuals or partnerships and were profit-making, whilst the remaining one-third were owned by non-profit-making bodies such as religious foundations.

So substantial changes were already taking place in America with regard to private psychiatric provision. As a result of this, and in an effort to clarify this role within the national picture of the American mental health system, Gibson points out that the National Institute of Mental Health and the National Association of Private Psychiatric Hospitals collaborated on a survey of admissions to private psychiatric hospitals in the United States.

The findings of the survey indicated that the private hospitals were admitting a large proportion of patients who had been referred by psychiatrists or other doctors, and who had serious psychiatric disorders such as schizophrenia or depressive disorders, that these patients were treated by psychotherapy or drug therapy (or both) and 90 per cent were discharged within 12 weeks. It also showed that the staff-patient ratios were on the whole higher in private psychiatric hospitals than in other mental health facilities, with the highest ratio in the private, non-profit-making hospitals.

On the basis of these findings, Gibson argued that the private psychiatric hospitals already had an advantage over other types of facility for a number of reasons. First, they were specialist and could therefore concentrate on the service they were giving the patients, whereas in other hospitals psychiatry would be one of many services which were provided. Second, because of this emphasis he claimed that the hospital would necessarily become 'a therapeutic instrument in its own right'. Finally, he claimed that rather than adversely affecting the quality of the service provided, the reliance on revenues from such services to patients could, in fact, stimulate good management. At the same time he acknowledged (1978, p. 20) a number of constraints on the psychiatric services provided by state hospitals and community mental health centres where he says that 'physical space, facilities for activities and specialised treatment services are often limited'.

This, together with deinstitutionalisation programmes imposed by politicians, he says, caused an erosion of resources with cost-cutting being a higher priority than the needs of the patients themselves. However, in spite of these comments, Gibson acknowledged that many state programmes were excellent and that enhancement in general terms could come with greater collaboration.

> At this juncture there is no reason to believe that one type of facility is in all respects superior to another. Each has its strengths depending on the mission and characteristics of the institution. For this reason, a pluralistic approach is in order and will probably continue indefinitely (1978, p. 19).

Essentially therefore, what Gibson argued in the mid to late 1970s was that ownership of mental health facilities did not matter all that much. However, somewhat more cautionary comments have since been made by other writers such as Dorwat and Schlesinger (1984). In their reappraisal of the move towards private mental health care, they suggest that there are a number of implications of this shift, the result of which is that ownership does matter because it affects the organisational behaviour of these facilities.

Like Gibson (1978) they attribute the growth in private psychiatric hospitals partly to an increased need for psychiatric beds to arising from the state policy of deinstitutionalisation. They also see it as a reclamation of territory rather than a complete innovation, and state (1984, p. 960) that 'the contemporary share of private psychiatric hospital beds under for-profit ownership is not unusually high by historical standards'. Also (1984, p. 963) that:

> the recent growth in for-profit ownership may be more accurately characterised as a recovery from past declines rather than as a fundamental shift in the delivery of in-patient psychiatric care.

They argue that these ownership-related trends do have important implications for mental health policy and it is this impact upon which they concentrate in three specific areas.

The first is how ownership impacts on access to care. Here, although they acknowledge the suggestion that private facilities 'screen out' patients who might be very costly to treat, they dismiss this proposition as being too vague and unsupported by relevant data. However, they do suggest that screening of this sort may take place on the basis of the patient's own ability to pay.

Second, they ask the question whether profit increases efficiency and changes the quality of care? This is another problematic area because it necessitates the measurement of quality which in itself has many variables. They cite the most common of these as being staff-patient ratios as an indicator of quality of care and highlight that studies have shown that staff resources are more generous in the private sector. In spite of this, they do not accept that the profit motive leads necessarily to more efficient care and contend that cost differences between the private and public sectors here are fairly minimal and in any case smaller than any differences in the quality of care.

Finally they explore what they call the 'fiduciary relationship between a facility and the community where it is located' (1984, p. 964).

In this respect, they claim that ownership makes a big impact because there appears to be far less willingness to provide a service like this to the locality unless there is sufficient likelihood of reimbursement and this creates a big difference between those who administer the private and the non-private facilities.

In spite of these cautionary comments, they acknowledge that the evidence they present is not definitive and leaves many unanswered questions. Unwilling to commit themselves about whether the private for-profit sector offers better care, they conclude by saying that:

> [t]he rapid expansion of proprietary ownership in mental health care and the simultaneous growth of psychiatric care in non-profit short-term general hospitals are very likely transforming both the way care is delivered and the fundamental structure of the mental health care system. We know enough to be concerned by these changes but as yet, too little to design effective policy responses (1984, p. 964).

In the same year that Dorwat and Schlesinger made these comments, a conference sponsored by the Tennessee Department of Mental Health was held, the purpose of which was to try to 'assess the organisation and financing of public and private mental health services and forecast future trends'. O'Connor (1984, p. 877) describes the conference as being dominated by concern over 'the rapid rise of the for-profit multihospital chains, the public sector's siege mentality, and the validity of applying free market principles to the mental health field'.

Concerns were voiced particularly over what was termed the 'aggressive' expansion of the proprietary world coupled with enormous suspicion of for-profit health care providers which were often seen as indicative of 'American ambivalence towards capitalism and socialised medicine'.

It was generally agreed that in America mental health was very big business. (At the time of O'Connor's 1984 article it was estimated that one-fifth of all United States spending on health care was on mental health care.) For instance, this could include a large business or a government agency buying mental health insurance for 10,000 employees at one time and yet it was remarked on that nothing existed to ensure the quality of care that such potential patients might receive.

It was generally agreed that there should be methods of ensuring accountability and ways of showing patients as consumers any differences which might exist between services and how they may be affected by them. The inherent problem in this area however, is that often the chronically mentally ill are tremendously vulnerable and cannot make informed decisions about the quality of their care. In the light of this it was proposed (O'Connor 1984, p. 879) that the state government should intercede on behalf of such people and promote information about this type of care with the ultimate intention of fostering competition amongst providers.

These then were the sorts of questions being raised in the United States regarding the move towards greater privatisation in the mental health care field up to the mid 1980s. Subsequent literature towards the end of the 1980s, when there had been a span of time allowing for reflection, appears to focus more strongly on the implications of this shift, and it can be illustrated by reference to the following literature.

In their 1988 paper for the *American Journal of Psychiatry*, Dorwat and Schlesinger give an overview of this trend together with implications for the future. In it they acknowledge that there is a need for further research to be carried out to assess the full implications of the move to for-profit privatisation, most particularly in four areas – those of access, quality, costs and appropriateness of care. They accept that whilst much of the concern to date is speculative, it is nonetheless worthy of note and produce a table of what they believe are commonly held assumptions in respect of for-profit and non-profit psychiatric facilities (see Table 3.1).

In respect of the main areas over which they express concern they concentrate on the first three in the following way. In terms of access there is the potential for imbalances based on ability to pay or funding and suggest (1988, p. 549) that there is definite evidence of selectivity on this basis from studies which have been carried out. Second, in terms of quality, they reiterate the fact that whilst this is arguably the most important, it is also the most difficult to measure in mental health care. From what little data they have, the suggestion is that there is little difference between private and public sector facilities, but this does acknowledge that there are no nationwide comparisons of costs among differently owned mental health facilities.

In their summing up, they address the issue of what they call 'community versus corporate responsibility'. In doing so, they concentrate heavily on the issue of motivation and the provision of mental health care. In the case of

Table 3.1   Common assumptions and characteristics in comparisons of for-profit and non-profit ownership of psychiatric facilities

For-profit	Non-profit
Owned and controlled by investors	Owned by non-profit corporation or trust controlled by volunteer board of directors
Mission usually stated in terms of growth	Mission often stated in terms of charity, quality or community service
Access restricted by ability to pay privately	Access not dependent on form of reimbursement but limited by insurance coverage
Quality under pressures of profit motive defined by consumer preferences	Quality often determined by professional values and also standards: treatment sometimes excessive
Increased costs due to higher charges, use of ancillary services, overheads and need to generate profits	Increased costs due to less efficiency, more professional staff, subsidisation of teaching and research
Less responsiveness to community needs	Priority to community service obligations
Treatment of different diagnostic mix of patients	Treatment of sicker and more chronically ill patients
Broader access to capital from equity, retained earnings, debt, etc.	Capital resources restricted coming from contributions, grants, bond debt
Profits subject to corporate tax	Exempt from federal and state tax

Source: table reproduced from Dorwat and Schlesinger, 1988, p. 549.

American community hospitals, they have traditionally been looked on as providers of a service for the 'public good', and receive tax-exempt status for this and therefore, Dorwat and Schlesinger (1988, p. 550) suggest that '[h]ospitals responding to financial incentives to maximise profits may be less likely to respond to local community needs than are tax-exempt institutions'.

They conclude that financial concerns must realistically be highly influential in providing the motivating force behind private for-profit psychiatric care, but at the same time say that it is not possible to generalise about this and that there is a need for further research.

Subsequent literature on this shows that research did take place in relation to for-profit and non-profit psychiatric provision in the United States and it is the findings of these upon which we will now concentrate with the purpose of determining whether previously speculative concerns are borne out by this.

This literature encompasses first, a 1990 study of the development of a medical-psychiatric programme within the private sector, and second a 1993 study of the relative performance of for-profit (in investor-owned systems) and non-profit psychiatric hospitals.

The study, carried out by Bruns and Stoudemire (1990), follows the development of a private, profit-making psychiatric unit allied to a general hospital in Nebraska intended to provide both medical and psychiatric services to the older population living in central and south Omaha, and (1990, p. 137):

> outlines the organisation and development of such a private unit and discusses the various medical, administrative, political and financial considerations that must be evaluated in planning for the successful operation of medical-psychiatric units within the private sector.

The authors primarily outline what they consider to be the potential problems affecting the success of setting up this sort of unit. These are first, the cost of treating patients who might have a lengthy stay in hospital; second the problem of reimbursement for those patients without adequate medical cover; third, the fact that treating the particular type of patients who would be admitted to this type of facility would be time-consuming and 'cost-inefficient'; and fourth, that it would in all probability be necessary, in the interests of feasibility, to keep a tight control on access to such a facility. They admit this may not sit as easily with the medical profession as it might with the directorship.

Prior to setting up this particular facility, Bruns and Stoudemire (1990) describe the process of carrying out an assessment in order to decide whether it was a viable proposition. On the basis of their findings it was decided that it should go ahead and they cite the following as being the primary reasons for this:

1   accelerated growth of the geriatric population;

2   increased growth in multiple illnesses in the older age-group;

3   declining or restricted resources in current health care;

4   high concentration of elderly patients in the immediate area;

5   expected expansion in the size of the market;

6   hospital well situated to meet the needs of the population.

On this basis it was suggested (1990, p. 138) that:

> there was an apparent unmet need for patients needing active medical/surgical treatment and psychiatric treatment simultaneously. Furthermore, it showed that this level of care could most likely be best provided within the medical facility ... Therefore, it was determined that a blend of medical and psychiatric approaches and techniques would be most effective.

One of the initial concerns when setting up the facility was that there should be clearly defined admission criteria. This was felt to be important both from a medical and financial point of view first because of the wish to minimise what were called 'the potential for denials of stay' (1990, p. 139) and second, because it was felt important that patients accepted into the unit should be capable of fully responding to and participating in their treatment. This gives some indication that selectivity was considered important at the outset. Allied to this was the concern over defining certain types of patients who should be excluded on the basis of exceeding the amount of medical care that could be provided.

In their summary, Bruns and Stoudemire state that the biggest problems in setting up this type of facility are those of costs and financial feasibility, particularly as they were looking to provide for more elderly patients in this particular hospital, who would necessarily command greater expense outlay than would similar, younger (and fitter) patients. As such, they indicate that private psychiatric units such as this are not potential 'moneyspinners', but nor should they be considered to be a total loss, financially. They state that it is possible that the financial problems such units potentially pose can be mitigated by (1990, p. 145):

> stringent and ongoing utilisation review, aggressive discharge planning, and an effort to achieve a case mix of shorter-stay/longer-stay admissions as well as a mix of both private and Medicare patients.

The primary indications from this example appear to support the previously speculative concerns made about access to private psychiatric care in terms of motivation being based to a great extent on fiscal considerations. Before we consider these questions further, we will look finally at the McCue and Clements (1993) study which analyses the differences between 42 matched pairs of for-profit and non-profit psychiatric hospitals from 1986 to 1990.

At the outset, McCue and Clements (1993, p. 77) acknowledge the concerns which have previously been expressed in relation to private for-profit hospitals in terms of the effect that pressure to achieve financial goals will have on access to and cost of care. As such they state that:

> [s]ince the financial goal of these hospitals is to maximise the wealth of shareholders, they have incentives to price their services aggressively, select profitable patients and keep expenses low.

As such their study seeks to ascertain whether the for-profit and non-profit hospitals differ in terms of revenue, price, expenses and what they call 'other performance measures'.

In order to control for market variables which might necessarily affect the performances to be measured, the 42 hospitals were matched, if possible first by location, seven hospitals being in the same county. Second, if this were not possible, they were matched on the basis of being in a 'standard metropolitan area' (1993, p. 78). McCue and Clements used 33 such hospitals. Finally where the first two criteria could not be matched, the hospitals were matched on the basis of having a similar wage index in their catchment area and two were used in this category. Having done this, the specific issues which were researched were first, operational performance and productivity, described by McCue and Clements as including occupancy rate and length of stay. Second came profitability and payer mix, including discharges per bed. Third were revenue and expenses and finally capital structure.

Based on their findings, McCue and Clements (1993, p. 81) conclude that '[i]n today's health care environment, cost control for mental health services is becoming a major goal of employers and insurers'. Their research focuses on four main findings which are as follows. First, they found that the for-profit hospitals had a higher net patient revenue per day and per discharge than did the non-profit hospitals. This they felt could be the result of either higher prices or a different 'payer mix' (mode of funding a bed) in the for-profit hospitals. Second, they found that the for-profit hospitals had lower salary expenses, a fact which they attributed to a reduction of staffing levels, either because it was possible that the for-profit hospitals were selecting less complex cases resulting in lower costs, or they felt it may have been a result of the fact that 'the greater number of hospitals owned by the for-profit systems may have enabled them to develop economies in staffing'.

The third main focus of their findings was in the area of routine care and ancillary services. Here, no significant differences were found. Finally, in terms of the capital structure of these respective hospitals, the for-profit hospitals were found to have on the whole much better facilities in terms of buildings and equipment which was a result of the fact that they had much greater access to debt capital because most were members of large for-profit organisations.

In conclusion, McCue and Clements suggest (1993, p. 82) that if the non-profit hospitals wish to compete fully with the for-profit ones, they too would need to upgrade their facilities, but the fact they have high salary costs and poor profitability necessarily restricts this and therefore 'nonprofit inpatient psychiatric hospitals may be at risk of closing or changing behaviour to emulate the more financially successful for-profit systems'.

Summary

What has been outlined in this chapter is first, an explanation of the growth of private psychiatric health care both in the United Kingdom and the United States and second, an investigation by way of the most current literature available, into the main issues and concerns which have been voiced in relation to this move. The question ultimately is, does ownership affect the nature of the service being provided?

Both in the United Kingdom and the United States, there have been recent expansions of the private provision of psychiatric services attributed to similar factors. In the United States, this gap in the market has been explained by Gibson (1978), Dorwat and Schlesinger (1984 and 1988) and others as having been the result of an increase in the prevalence of psychiatric illness, and a growth in the purchasing, on a large scale, of this sort of specific health cover or insurance, not just by individuals, but also by large companies on behalf of their employees. Thus, it has become a lucrative corner of the health care market. This expansion has also been explained as being due in part to a process of deinstitutionalisation, backed by the government.

Similarly, in Britain, there have been moves towards deinstitutionalisation of the mentally ill, but in a country where the National Health Service predominates, this move has been slower in producing the alternative of private psychiatric care in place of public sector provision. In fact, in the United Kingdom, it has been American companies such as Partnerships in Care who have sought this attractive business opportunity, based on their experience abroad. In Britain, changes in the provision of psychiatric care have most often resulted in complaints about the lack of beds which now exist, which has been documented by Watson (1994). This lack has been particularly marked in the area of medium security. Therefore, the more recent moves towards privatisation of psychiatric services in the United Kingdom are not all that surprising in the current climate. What we are now witnessing is in some small way a mirroring of the American experience in this sphere of health care, although it obviously differs substantially in respect of the funding of beds.[1] We might expect therefore, that with the primacy of the National Health Service and inherent suspicion regarding privatisation in general, that the British response to this issue would differ from that of our American counterparts. However, this assumption would essentially be incorrect.

The literature shows that although this process has been ongoing in the United States for approximately 30 years,[2] their concerns, first speculative and then supported by research, are similar to the concerns which are now being voiced in relation to the move towards private psychiatric care in the United Kingdom. Those concerns have their basis in the question of whether ownership of psychiatric services actually matters, and revolve around four main issues, those of access, profit, quality of care and community needs. To summarise, each of these will be addressed.

Access

The issue of access and selectivity has been one of the major areas of concern generated by the literature which has been reviewed. In the United Kingdom, it was suggested at the outset that there may be financial pressures upon private psychiatric hospitals to keep empty beds to a minimum and thus there may be the possibility of such facilities admitting patients for whom their services are inappropriate. In the United States, Dorwat and Schlesinger (1984) initially suggested that screening of patients on the basis of their ability to pay might be a problem, a fact which they reiterate in a later publication, and these suggestions regarding the possibilities for manipulation of access to profit-making hospitals was to some extent borne out by the study carried out by Bruns and Stoudemire (1990). Here, during the setting up of a psychiatric unit of this type, tight controls on access and the use of admission criteria were focused on, in order to achieve what was called a 'good mix' of patients to ensure profitability and fiscal feasibility.

In the same way, questions need to be asked regarding whether these sorts of policies operate in relation to American-owned private psychiatric hospitals in Britain and whether the same pressures force a similar process of selectivity. In this respect the later chapters of this study will focus on a comparative admissions study in order to determine on what basis, if any, selectivity operates and how access may differ between public and private sector medium secure psychiatric provision within the United Kingdom.

Profit

The second area outlined is that of profit. It has been suggested that in the United Kingdom private psychiatric care is relatively expensive and beds are normally funded by the Local Health Authority from which the patient originates. This happens if there is no bed locally, if the patient is deemed to be 'unmanageable' in terms of behaviour and therefore very costly, if the Home Office requests a bed or sometimes if a patient may be long-term, as local secure hospitals, (RSUs) cannot normally cater for patients likely to be hospitalised for more than two years. In this sense, referral to a private psychiatric facility is a good business opportunity for the accepting facility. Does this mean that profit is more important than the quality of service? This is something about which there has been much speculation in the United States. Gibson (1978) felt that reliance on revenue stimulated good management, but other writers have been more cautious. Dorwat and Schlesinger (1988) felt that profit was a motive in any of the American facilities because even the nonprofit-making hospitals would get tax-exemption by servicing the local community. Bruns and Stoudemire (1990) similarly show how important the notion of costs, reimbursement, etc. are when considering the feasibility of establishing new facilities of this type. Also McCue and Clements (1993) reiterate the importance of the issue of profit in their comparative study which showed that the for-profit hospitals in their study had higher patient revenues because they deliberately took a mix of patients with the intention of affecting their total funding. This suggests that realistically fiscal considerations do affect the organisational behaviour of profit-making hospitals. What is uncertain is whether it is actually detrimental, beneficial or neither. This is also an area which requires further research.

Quality

All the literature reviewed has suggested that one of the most important concerns in relation to the provision of private mental health care is that of the quality of care being provided and how it might be effectively monitored.

Gibson (1978, p. 20) points out that in his opinion, the quality of care being provided by such facilities could be described as 'excellence which goes far beyond simply meeting needs at an acceptable level of quality'. He emphasises this level of quality by referring to the fact that there is a more direct relationship with the patients, because the hospitals are necessarily specialised in this field. This, he says, creates an organised environment which is an advantage in terms of therapy. He also makes the point that the reliance on revenue makes private hospitals more conscious of the quality of the service they are providing. He accepts however that staff/patient ratios (very often used as an indicator of quality) are highest in the private nonprofit hospitals.

Dorwat and Schlesinger (1984) too found that private nonprofit facilities had what they call 'more favourable' staffing ratios than other types of facility, but said that these differences were fairly minimal. Apart from this, they are far more reserved about the issue of quality of care in the private sector than Gibson because:

> [t]he debate over whether the profit motive is more likely to encourage increased efficiency or reductions in the quality of care cannot be resolved without accurate measures of quality of care (1984, p. 962).

This, they say is very difficult to do in mental health care, data on staff-to-patient ratios being the only commonly cited structural measures. They also mention, like Gibson, the issue of organisational efficiency, which Gibson claimed was increased by the profit motive. Dorwat and Schlesinger (1984, p. 961) however have this to say:

> [t]he hypothesis that the profit motive improves organisational efficiency is difficult to test without more complete measures of case mix and quality of care.

It is generally agreed that what is most important is that there should be a method for ensuring proper accountability in terms of quality of care and this concern is most aptly stated by O'Connor (1984, p. 878) who cites Schlesinger at the 1984 Tennessee Conference on mental health as saying:

> [i]t is amazing to me that there is nothing in the research literature that explores how terms of contracts affect efficacy and quality of care or the types of patient served. We should attempt to identify contract features that influence the role of the private provider.

Although there is even less research literature on private mental health provision in the United Kingdom, that which exists suggests the concerns which are currently prevalent regarding the move to privatisation in the United Kingdom are very similar to those identified in the American literature.

It has been established that although private psychiatric provision is relatively new in the United Kingdom, there are already points in relation to that provision which demand further research. Market forces have been seen to be prevalent in terms of the fact that referrals to private psychiatric hospitals do receive prompt attention, but this method of referral is such that it is most often the patient's local health authority, as the funding body, which is the 'customer' in this contract and not the patient, and the resultant fact that the referral is often from an authority many miles away from the private hospital, makes it all the more difficult to address the issue of the quality of care being provided. Factors other than dislocation also affect the quality of the care provided in this way. Issues such as continuation of care and follow-up after discharge also pose a problem and these are all issues which need to be addressed by further research. However, as Dorwat and Schlesinger found in the United States, it is similarly difficult to assess quality in the United Kingdom and gaining access to the relevant data can be most difficult. This difficulty and how it impacts upon this research will be discussed further at the end of this chapter. Finally we address the last area of identifiable concern which is that of community needs.

Community Needs

The issue of community needs and how privatisation of psychiatric care impacts upon this is discussed most extensively by Dorwat and Schlesinger (1984). They found less willingness in the private sector to provide psychiatric services for the local community unless there was sufficient reimbursement. This indicates very clearly a process of selectivity based upon fiscal motives.

In their later article on the same subject they reiterate this, (1988, p. 550) but also make the point that albeit in a different way, community hospitals in the United States are to some extent motivated to provide a service to the community because for doing this, they receive tax exemptions which the private sector does not.

The issue of funding has also been outlined as relevant in the United Kingdom and this does have an impact on the issue of service to the community. The private psychiatric hospital here also does not, on the face of it, work as a community hospital taking as it does referrals from regional psychiatric units all over the country. The impetus for accepting referrals includes the fact that a bed must be paid for, whether by the funding health authority of the patient, or by private means and as such the private hospital fits into the psychiatric picture of care on a national basis rather than a regional one. Therefore the implications as far as community needs are concerned are the same in the United Kingdom as have been elucidated by the American writers.

Conclusion

This literature review has made it evident that in relation to the privatisation of psychiatric health care both in America and subsequently in the United Kingdom, four issues are of prime concern and merit further study. These have been identified as the issues of access, profit, community needs and quality of care. This study, which in chapters 5, 6 and 7 will focus mainly on access to public and private sector psychiatric hospitals in the United Kingdom, intended at the outset to look also into the respective regimes of both types of facility, and as such some research into all four areas may theoretically have been possible. However, after data had been collected on the admission and discharge of patients at Stockton Hall (the private psychiatric hospital which forms the basis of this study), a change in the management structure of the hospital necessitated a renegotiation of the access which had been granted in respect of patient medical files. During this process it was made clear that data other than that already accessed, would not be made available. This made it impossible to study the sort of regime currently in operation at Stockton Hall and thus negated the possibility of further research into areas which lay directly outside that gleaned from the admission and discharge data to which I had access. It is on this basis therefore, that the study was carried out. It will concentrate on the issue of access to public and private sector psychiatric care although we will also consider how issues such as profit and community needs impact upon patient admissions and address the question of the operation of selectivity.

The next chapter explains some of the legal and medical issues involved in the provision of psychiatric care, including its regulation by the Mental Health Act 1983 and how this legislation deals with people who are deemed to require psychiatric hospitalisation in conditions of security. It explains the procedures necessary for sectioning under the Act and the passage into secure care of those deemed by the law, to require it.

Notes

1 It should be noted than an entirely accurate comparison cannot truly be made between the two countries as there is no United States equivalent of the United Kingdom public sector psychiatric hospital. Therefore, any comparisons which are made are done on the basis of a comparison between public and private sector provision in the United Kingdom and private non-profit and for-profit provision in the United States. This is still a useful comparison to make.
2 By this I mean specifically in relation to psychiatric provision and not in relation to the American health care system in general.

4 Mental Health Care and the Law

This chapter provides an outline of the legal procedures involved in a person being considered under the Mental Health Act 1983 for psychiatric admission. Included in this will be the defences for a person who cannot be said to be responsible for his actions, (insanity and diminished responsibility) when tried for a criminal offence, as well as the cases where a person is responsible but requires treatment – which must be brought to the judge's notice at the time of sentencing. The sentences available to the court will also be examined as will a description of the existing psychiatric facilities and the process of discharge by reference to the Mental Health Review Tribunal. Some explanation of these procedures are necessary in order fully to understand the process by which patients come to be held, under the Mental Health Act 1983, in conditions of security and the factors which influence this process.

Mental Disorder and the Law

The procedures under which the courts may place a criminal offender in psychiatric provision are contained in the Mental Health Act 1983 (MHA '83). A useful starting point to an analysis of these provisions is an outline of the legal categories of mental disorder and a comparison with medical categories. Having defined mental disorder in terms of the Act, the legal procedures may be outlined. The law perceives two categories of mentally ill offender, those who cannot be said to be responsible for their actions (who will plead insanity or diminished responsibility when tried for a criminal offence) and those who are responsible but require treatment (which must be brought to the judge's attention at the time of sentencing). A person may also be found to be unfit to stand trial or to plead, in which case the provisions of the Criminal Procedure (Insanity) Act 1964 and the Criminal Procedure (Insanity and Fitness to Plead) Act 1991 will be relevant. These defences will be examined in greater detail together with the sentencing options of the court and the provisions for transferring persons serving prison sentences to psychiatric facilities.

The Legal Categories of Mental Disorder

Section 1(2) of the MHA '83 defines mental disorder as 'mental illness, arrested or incomplete development of the mind, psychopathic disorder and any other disorder or disability of mind'.

The Act distinguishes between major and minor disorders and therefore, for a person to become a patient, he must be suffering from either one of the major disorders – mental illness or severe mental impairment, or a minor disorder – psychopathic disorder or mental impairment. It will be helpful to examine each of the categories in turn.

Mental illness Mental illness has not been defined by statute and so has been left open to interpretation by the various medical personnel who must diagnose it. The Butler Committee (1975) defined it as a 'disorder which has not always existed in the patient but has developed as a condition overlying the sufferer's usual personality', which coincides with those medical practitioners who would link organic disturbances (psychoses) with the term 'illness', whereas other conditions are not illnesses but extreme variations in personality from a hypothetical norm. Some doctors, however, would assert that neuroses (such as anxieties, hysteria, phobias, obsessions, reactive depression, etc.), or at least some of them may also be classed as an illness as they involve an obvious departure from normal health. The most useful definition so far was suggested by the Northern Ireland Review Committee on Mental Health Legislation (1981, p. 1) which contended that mental illness was:

> a state of mind of a permanent or temporary (but not merely transient) nature in which the individual exhibits such disordered thinking, perceiving or emotion as impairs judgement of the situation to the extent that he requires care, treatment or training in his own interests or in the interests of other persons.

Psychopathic disorder Section 1(2) of the MHA '83 defines psychopathic disorder as:

> a persistent disorder or disability of mind (whether or not including significant impairment of intelligence) which results in abnormally aggressive or seriously irresponsible conduct on the part of the person concerned.

The idea of a specific disorder which is particularly related to antisocial behaviour has been established for some time. The concept has been criticised particularly in its application to criminal offenders. Here the question is whether or not this group of offenders should be singled out for special treatment as it would appear to be a circular argument to conclude that a person is disordered because he commits crimes and then conclude that his disorder should partially excuse his crimes. There is further practical difficulty in sending psychopaths for treatment as few of them respond to the conventional forms of treatment. Because they are often difficult or troublesome patients, they are not always welcomed by hospital staff. This results in the label 'psychopath' doing an offender more harm than good as few hospitals will be prepared to admit and treat them. There is then the difficulty of proving that such a patient is safe to release. In these circumstances such an offender may be sentenced to prison for the longest period that a court has power to grant because of the perception of dangerousness.

Mental impairment and severe mental impairment These provisions are relevant to people who are mentally handicapped. The MHA '83, s1(2) defined severe mental impairment as:

> a state of arrested or incomplete development of mind which includes severe impairment of intelligence and social functioning and is associated with abnormally aggressive or seriously irresponsible conduct on the part of the person concerned.

Mental impairment is defined in the same section as:

> a state of arrested or incomplete development of mind (not amounting to severe impairment) which includes significant impairment of intelligence and social functioning and is associated with abnormally aggressive or seriously irresponsible conduct on the part of the person concerned.

Therefore, for powers of long detention including hospital orders and transfers from prison, the patient's mental handicap must be associated with psychopathic behaviour.

The Medical Categories of Mental Disorder

The classifications of mental disorder are manifold and it is difficult to establish any general consensus of medical opinion. However, Prins (1995) outlines the categories thus:

a) *Functional psychoses* These would be severe mental disorders with no underlying organic dysfunction and would include the affective disorders such as manic depressive illness and also schizophrenia.

b) *Neuroses* Less severe in nature and would include mild depression, anxiety states and hysteria.

c) *Mental disorder* Resulting from infection, disease, metabolic disturbance or trauma. These would include encephalitis, Huntington's Chorea, endocrine disorders, brain tumours and epilepsy.

d) *Mental disorder* Caused by the ageing process such as presenile and senile dementia.

e) *Personality disorder* Including psychosexual disorders and psychopathy.

f) *Alcohol and other drug addictions.*

g) *Mental subnormality or handicap, where a person's IQ is estimated to be below 70.*

Mental Disorder as a Defence

Insanity The special verdict of 'not guilty by reason of insanity' is the result of the conflicting notions that whilst a person who is mentally disordered and not responsible for his actions should not be punished with the full force of the criminal law, he should also not be left at large in society. The accepted formulation of the legal concept of insanity was given by the judiciary in response to questions from the House of Lords in *M'Naghten's Case* (1843) where it was held that:

> to establish a defence on the grounds of insanity, it must be clearly proved that, at the time of committing the act, the party accused was labouring under such a defect of reason, from disease of the mind, as not to know the nature and quality of the act [he] was doing, or, if [he] did know it, that [he] did not know that it was wrong.

In *R v Kemp* (1957) Devlin, J. defined 'mind' as meaning the mental faculties of reason, memory and understanding. In the House of Lords decision in *R v Sullivan* (1983) it was said that:

> if the effect of a disease was to impair those faculties so severely as to have either of the consequences referred to in the latter part of the rules, it mattered not whether the impairment was organic, as in epilepsy, or functional, or intermittent, provided that it subsisted at the time of the commission of the act.

However, non-insane automatism could still be possible where a temporary impairment was brought about by an external factor such as a blow to the head or the therapeutic administration of drugs. Thus, an epileptic may be insane where a diabetic is either innocent or guilty (if he knows that a combination of insulin, food and alcohol may make him aggressive or uncontrolled and was reckless as to this effect).

The Butler Committee (1975) proposed that there should be a special verdict of 'not guilty on evidence of mental disorder' in situations where the mental disorder will negate the state of mind required for the commission of the particular offence. More radically, it proposed that the defence should be available whenever the accused was suffering from severe mental illness or severe mental handicap – with no requirement to establish a causal link between the disorder and the offence.

This second aspect of the Committee's recommendations has never been implemented and whilst it is attractive to those who do not believe in trying the mentally ill at all it provides no solution to the question of criminal responsibility or liability. Insanity has been interpreted by the judiciary in the light of its acknowledgement that the purpose of the special verdict is not to protect or excuse the defendant, but to protect society from any recurrence of such dangerous conduct. Under the Criminal Procedure (Insanity) Act 1964, s5(1), once the verdict has been reached, the defendant would be detained in a hospital specified by the Home Secretary, with the same status as a restriction order patient. In practice, the only time an insanity plea was used was when indefinite detention in a Special Hospital was preferable to the prison sentence – which could only be when the charge was murder, the fixed penalty for which is life imprisonment. The 1964 Act has now been amended by the Criminal Procedure (Insanity and Unfitness to Plead) Act 1991, which came into force on 1 January 1992. Section 1 of this Act provides that a jury must not return a verdict of not guilty by reason of insanity except on the evidence of two or more medical practitioners, one of whom is approved under the Mental Health Act 1983.

Under section 3 of the 1991 Act, the court will be able to choose between a range of orders, bearing in mind the circumstances of the case, the severity of the offence and the needs of the defendant. A restriction order is only compulsory where the accused has been found to have committed an offence for which the sentence is fixed by law, i.e. murder, or where it is considered necessary to protect the public from serious harm. One of the aims of the new Act was to alleviate the severe consequences of the insanity verdict, which in the past had resulted in many people preferring to plead guilty to crimes for which they were not really responsible.

Diminished responsibility Diminished responsibility may be used as a defence to the charge of murder. If successful it will reduce the offence to manslaughter. According to the Homicide Act 1957 s2, the accused must be suffering from 'such abnormality of mind (whether arising from a condition of arrested development of mind or any inherent cause or induced by disease or injury) as substantially impaired his responsibility'.

Since the case of *R v Byrne* (1960) the phrase 'abnormality of mind' has been widely accepted as meaning 'a state so different from that of ordinary human beings that a reasonable man would term it abnormal'.

The Criminal Law Revision Committee 1980 would prefer the present criterion to be replaced with the concept of mental disorder as defined in the MHA '83. The second requirement of 'impaired responsibility' does not refer to the legal concept of responsibility which would make the defence similar to insanity, but a question of moral turpitude which cannot be answered expertly by either doctors or lawyers. The Butler Committee suggested that this difficulty could be overcome if the mandatory life sentence for murder were to be abolished and sentencing left to judicial discretion. This would mean that a statutory formulation to define when murder becomes manslaughter would be avoided.

Unfitness to plead At the time a person is brought for trial he may be found unfit to plead to the indictment under s4 of the Criminal Procedure (Insanity) Act 1964. As a result of this, the courts have evolved tests in order to determine whether the defendant is indeed unfit to plead. To establish this, courts might ask the following questions: is the defendant able to understand the charge?; is he able to challenge jurors?; is he able to instruct counsel?; is he able to follow the evidence?; if he is capable of all these things he has a right to be tried if he so wishes, even if he is not capable of acting in his own best interests.

The Criminal Procedure (Insanity and Unfitness to Plead) Act 1991 establishes that a person is not to be found unfit to plead except on the evidence of two or more medical practitioners, at least one of whom must be approved by the Secretary of State as having special expertise in the field of mental disorder as defined by the Mental Health Act 1983.

The 1991 Act also allows the court to retain its power to postpone consideration of the question of fitness until any time before the opening of the case for the defence. This allows the case for the prosecution to be tested and if there is insufficient evidence, the defendant can be acquitted without the need to consider fitness. It also enables the court to consider the intention of the accused (i.e. the *mens rea*), where appropriate.

Unfitness to trial Under the 1991 Act if a jury decides the accused is unfit to stand trial, the court is required to conduct a 'trial of the facts'. This involves the jury examining all the evidence of the case including forensic, scientific and witness evidence in order to determine whether the accused committed the alleged act or omission 'beyond reasonable doubt', although the *mens rea* of the accused is not taken into account. Once a decision is reached, the jury may make a 'finding' that the accused committed the act or was responsible for the omission – which is a different legal concept to a conviction – or it may acquit and the accused will not be subject to any of the 1991 Act disposals. The Act further safeguards the rights of the accused by allowing the court to appoint a person to ensure that the legal representatives are instructed for his defence in the trial of the facts and it also contains provisions to clarify when the jury, which decides the question of fitness, may or may not be the same as the jury in the trial of the facts.

Sentencing

The courts have been provided with a broad range of non-penal disposals to consider when the question of sentencing a mentally disordered offender arises. There are five specifically psychiatric orders, two of which are psychiatric probation orders and guardianship orders. The other three psychiatric orders which are more relevant to this study are types of hospital order and will be considered in greater detail, as will the option of transfer from prison to hospital.

Hospital Orders

An ordinary hospital order can be made for any offence, except for those with a fixed penalty. In practice this means murder.

For a Crown Court to make a hospital order, it must have convicted the person of the offence, whereas Magistrates Courts may impose a hospital order on a mentally ill or severely impaired defendant without recording a conviction, provided they are satisfied that he did the act or omission charged. The MHA '83 contains two criteria which must be considered; the medical and judicial.

The medical criterion is that two doctors, one of whom must be approved, must state that the person is suffering from a mental illness, psychopathic disorder, severe mental impairment or mental impairment. According to the MHA '83, s37(2)(a), the disorder must be 'of a nature or degree which makes it appropriate to be detained in hospital for medical treatment', and in the case of psychopathic disorder and mild mental impairment, this treatment must be likely to alleviate or prevent a deterioration of the condition. The doctors must agree on at least one of the four forms of disorder. Interpretation of these provisions by the medical profession has amounted to them having a certain amount of scope to 'pick and choose' those people whom they wish to place in hospitals and those they would rather leave to the Prison Service. If a doctor wishes to recommend a hospital order for someone who is a sexual offender or a drug addict (who falls outside the definition of those people who can be the subject of a hospital order) he would have to give evidence of some specific psychiatric disorder or illness. The 'treatability' test may also be used in the same way, as psychiatrists have the discretion to say whether the patient's condition is treatable or not. A further element of choice is that a court cannot make a hospital order unless it has evidence, either from the doctor who would be in charge of the patient or a representative of the hospital, that a bed will be available for him within 28 days. (MHA'83, s37(4).

The judicial criterion is that once the court has the required medical evidence, it must make a choice between punishment and treatment, having regard to all the circumstances of the case, including the nature of the offence, the character and antecedents of the offender, the need to protect the public and to the other available methods of dealing with him (MHA'83, s37(2)(b).

Interim Hospital Orders

Courts also have the option under the MHA '83, s38 to make an interim hospital order. This is similar to an ordinary hospital order with respect to the medical evidence needed. The important difference is that the order lasts for a period specified by the court, up to a maximum of 12 weeks. The court can renew it for further periods of 28 days to a maximum of six months. Once it is at an end, a court has a completely free choice amongst the disposals available for the offence for which the defendant was convicted. This gives a court a chance to decide what measure would be most appropriate for the offender and to avoid the harsh consequences of a mistaken diagnosis.

Restriction Orders

A restriction order was an attempt to combine the advantages of a hospital order with the advantages of indefinite preventive detention. Under s4(1) MHA '83, this can only be made in the Crown Court and the evidence required by the court is the same as that required for an ordinary hospital order. A doctor must also attend to give evidence. The question of whether a restriction order is appropriate is ultimately one for the judge, although the hospital's opinion may be taken into account. The court must come to the conclusion that the restriction order is necessary to protect the public from serious harm and once the order is made, the burden placed upon the offender to justify his release is a weighty one. This type of order can be imposed for a definite period or without limit of time (MHA '83, s42(1). The length of stay is not determined by the gravity of the offence, but by the length of time it will take to treat the patient.

The Court of Appeal in *R v Gardiner* (1967) held that restriction orders should be made without limit of time unless the doctors could confidently predict recovery within a limited period. The Home Secretary can lift restrictions at any time provided he is satisfied that they are no longer necessary to protect the public from serious harm, after which the patient is treated as if he had been admitted under an ordinary hospital order on the day the restriction order ended (MHA '83, s42(5) & 42(1), except that he may apply to a Mental Health Review Tribunal within his first six months.

While restrictions last, the MHA '83, s41(3)(c) stipulates that the patient cannot be discharged or, according to s41(3)(d), transferred to another hospital or even given leave of absence without the Home Secretary's permission. If this is obtained, the Home Secretary or the Resident Medical Officer may recall him. In the case of the Home Secretary, this need not be within the usual six month time limit.

The crucial difference between an ordinary hospital order and a restriction order is that the latter continues indefinitely. While the restrictions last and the patient has not been discharged absolutely, there is no statutory requirement that the detention be reviewed periodically. There is no obligation to consider whether the criteria still apply.

However, a European case has forced a reconsideration of this situation. The case of *X v United Kingdom* (1981) makes it clear that if a patient no longer suffers from mental disorder of a nature or degree which makes detention in hospital appropriate, he can no longer be detained there no matter how dangerous.

The MHA '83, s41(6) now provides that the Responsible Medical Officer must examine the patient and report to the Home Secretary at such intervals as the latter may require, but no more frequently than once a year. As yet there is no provision for a formal renewal procedure.

Transfer from Prison to Hospital

Another way in which offenders may find themselves committed to psychiatric hospital is by transfer from prison. The Home Secretary can direct that offenders serving prison sentences, assessed by prison medical officers as being mentally disordered within the meaning of the MHA '83, can be transferred to hospital under s47. The Home Secretary must have reports from two doctors, one of whom must be approved, and the same criteria as for ordinary admission must then be fulfilled. According to MHA '83, s 47(1) the Home Secretary must consider the transfer 'expedient' having regard to the public interest and all the circumstances of the case. Transfer without restrictions under s47(2) has the same effect as an ordinary hospital order and is often chosen where the prisoner is coming to the end of his sentence, and may mean that he will be legally liable to remain in hospital beyond the time when he would have been released from prison. This type of patient may be released at any time and may apply to a tribunal even within the first six months. Restrictions are normally imposed if the sentence has some time to run, in which case they cease automatically at the end of the sentence (s50(2)).

The patient has the right to apply to the tribunal within the first six months, although this does not mean that the tribunal has the power to discharge if it finds that he is no longer a suitable case for treatment. Once again the RMO is obliged to make regular examinations.

Absolute Discharge

The Criminal Procedure (Insanity and Unfitness to Plead) Act 1991 gives the court the option to grant an absolute discharge in cases where no order is necessary. This is likely to be used where the offence is fairly trivial and the person does not need treatment or supervision.

Psychiatric Facilities

Once the decision has been made that an offender should be made the subject of a hospital order or transferred from prison to hospital, the choice of facilities to deal with this type of patient is very limited. Currently there are four types of psychiatric facility in the United Kingdom and patients are referred on the basis of which level of security they require. These are as follows:

a) the psychiatric ward of a general NHS hospital;

b) a Regional Secure Unit (RSU) in medium security;

c) an independent medium secure psychiatric hospital;

d) a Special Hospital in maximum security.

At this point it is pertinent to outline a little more closely the criteria for admission to a psychiatric hospital. This necessitates a discussion of the requirements of 'dangerousness' and 'treatability' which are relevant in the context of the later study discussed in relation to that cohort of patients admitted to a private secure hospital, previously having been identified as unmanageable elsewhere. It may also be useful to examine the Mental Health Review Tribunal procedure in order to gain an insight into the factors which are taken into account when deciding if a patient should no longer be the subject of a detention order.

Criteria for Admission and Release

The special criteria for admission to a psychiatric, rather than an ordinary hospital are that the offender must be seen as both 'dangerous' *and* 'treatable'. These issues will be the focus of the following discussion.

Treatability

The 'treatability' test is derived from the MHA '83, s3(2)(a), where it is said that the disorder must be 'of a nature or degree which makes it appropriate for medical treatment'.

In the case of mental illness, it is often obvious that medical treatment is appropriate, in that the mental illness can be perceived as being curable or at least amenable to treatment. However, in some cases, such as psychopathic disorder and mental impairment, treatability is more often an issue. Therefore according to s34(7) any treatment must 'be likely to alleviate or prevent a deterioration of the condition'.

Prins (1995) sees psychopathy as part of a spectrum of personality disorder with treatability dependent upon the category into which a person's condition falls. He gives these categories as being:

a) minor behaviour disorder;

b) serious personality disorder, including unusual and affectionless personalities';

c) 'pseudo-psychopathy', due to temporal lobe disease, brain damage or infection;

d) essential psychopathy.

It is his suggestion that the first three are very difficult and the fourth impossible to treat. He sees this as the 'dustbin' category to which all the most difficult and unresponsive patients are assigned. Blackburn (1993) studied psychopathic patients in Special Hospitals and confirms the variety of clinical features subsumed under this term and that treatment can include nursing care, habilitation and rehabilitation under medical supervision. Thus, as Gunn (1978) points out:

> it is difficult to argue that in hospitals of any kind, a structured environment is a medical strategy, it is simply a prerequisite for making sure that patients stay where they are told to stay.

A psychiatrist has the job of deciding whether a person has a mental illness of the type which comes within the ambit of the MHA 1983 and therefore, in terms of treatment, whether that individual can be considered for admission to the appropriate psychiatric facility.

Dangerousness

The second criterion for psychiatric hospitalisation is dangerousness. This arose from the provision in the National Health Service Act 1977 s4, which required the Secretary of State to provide Special Hospitals:

> for persons subject to detention under the Mental Health Act who, in his opinion, require treatment in conditions of special security on account of their dangerous, violent or criminal propensities.

Walker and McCabe (1973) suggest that dangerousness is not an objective quality, but an ascribed quality like trustworthiness. We feel justified in talking about a person as dangerous if he has indicated by word or deed that he is more likely than most people to do serious harm. They also suggest that harm in this context is likely to be interpreted as acts such as homicide, rape, mutilation or the promotion of destitution (serious theft or fraud). The Butler Committee (1975) also examined the question of dangerousness and commented that:

> [w]e have come to equate dangerousness with a tendency to cause serious physical injury or lasting psychological harm. Physical violence is, we think, what the public are most worried about, but the psychological damage which may be suffered by some victims of other crime is not to be underrated.

Scott (1974, p. 640) supplies a neat summary in which he comments that:

> dangerousness then is an unpredictable and untreatable tendency to inflict serious, irreversible injury or destruction, or to induce others to do so. Dangerousness can, of course, be directed against the self.

So although a definition of dangerousness is not difficult to find, assessment and prediction of dangerousness have caused much controversy. Scott encapsulates the relevant criteria for predicting dangerousness in this simple equation:

offender + victim + circumstances = offence

Although this definition is conceptually simple, it is still the application which makes prediction and assessment so difficult. At present, methods are not refined enough to distinguish accurately those who are dangerous from those who are not, although sometimes it is possible to establish certain common characteristics present in many long-term difficult to treat patients which could be effective indicators of their levels of dangerousness and amenability. These factors can also be instrumental in determining the place of diversion of patients deemed to be either dangerous, untreatable or even both. The same difficulties exist when predicting whether a patient is safe to be released. Inevitably doctors may feel the need to err on the side of caution. The public outcry which occurs when an ex-patient offends or re-offends is inevitably far greater than that which may occur in response to the prolonged detention of people who no longer 'need' to be kept in conditions of security. Prins (1995) discusses a number of case profiles which help to illustrate the application and difficulties associated with the concepts of dangerousness and treatability. His purpose was to highlight particularly those cases where the patient had been released from conditions of security, having been assessed as no longer dangerous, but then who re-offended and had to be readmitted. In outlining two such cases it is possible to offer some initial insight into the types of patient with which such facilities seek to deal.

His first example is that of Graham Young who was convicted of administering poison to his father, sister and a school friend in 1962. At his trial it was said that his behaviour was highly deliberate and dangerous and he was made the subject of a hospital order with restrictions on his discharge. Young was to spend nine years in Broadmoor before he was conditionally discharged in 1971. He then found employment as a storekeeper where he had access to noxious chemicals and soon began to administer these to his fellow employees. He was subsequently sentenced to life imprisonment.

His second example is that of Terence John Iliffe, who had been detained in Broadmoor following the murder of his wife. A similar conditional discharge was made after it was decided that he had only been a danger to his wife. Upon release, Iliffe married again and murdered his second wife. He too was sentenced to life imprisonment.

Cases like these indicate that some patients within psychiatric hospitals are those who have committed grave crimes, and are suffering from major mental disorders which are persistent, long-lived and difficult to treat. Chapter six looks more specifically at the diversion of long-term patients and at the problems these patients can pose in terms of gaining access to psychiatric care if they have been labelled as 'unmanageable'. What is finally pertinent in this section is to address the process of discharge itself by reference to the Mental Health Review Tribunal.

Mental Health Review Tribunals

Unrestricted Patients

If a patient is detained under an ordinary hospital order, he must not be discharged if:

a) he is suffering from mental illness, psychopathic disorder, severe mental impairment or mental impairment; or

b) the disorder is not of a nature or degree which makes it appropriate for him to be detained in a hospital for medical treatment; or

c) it is not necessary for the health or safety of the patient or for the protection of other persons that he should receive such treatment.

The tribunal does not however, have to discharge patients who are deemed to be untreatable. Most important, if any one of the criteria for releasing the patient exists, he must be released whether dangerous or not.

Restriction Order Patients

Exactly the same criteria for release are applicable as in the case of unrestricted patients. However, a person who has been sent to hospital fairly recently as a psychopath, after having committed a serious offence, will find it extremely difficult to convince the tribunal that he is no longer or never was a psychopath. The tribunal does have the power (MHA '83, s72(1)), to choose between an absolute and conditional discharge. It must grant an absolute discharge if satisfied that it is not appropriate for the patient to remain liable to recall to hospital for further treatment. Otherwise, it must discharge with conditions (s73(2)).

Prisoners Transferred with Restrictions

The tribunal must decide whether the patient ought to remain in hospital. At this point it may become a matter for the Home Secretary to decide whether a patient should be transferred back to prison, if that is where he originated. Otherwise release may be to the community. In cases such as this the tribunal must notify the Home Secretary whether the patient is entitled to an absolute or conditional discharge. In the case of a conditional discharge, under MHA '83, s74(1) the patient can be entitled to remain in hospital rather than being returned to prison. The criteria for admission and detention and those for discharge can be seen, therefore, to be very similar, although the emphasis at admission seems to be on dangerousness and treatability. On discharge, the issues have become 'requirement of treatment' and 'treatment for the protection of others or of himself'.

Having established these criteria, their importance in relation to patients admitted into public sector regional secure units or private medium secure provision will subsequently become more evident. The following chapter discusses the development of the regional secure unit and focuses specifically on a recent study into comparative admissions and discharges from two such facilities.

5 Access to Public Sector Psychiatric Care: A Study of Admissions to Two Regional Secure Units 1989–92

Chapter 3 suggested a number of problems in providing private sector psychiatric hospitals. It outlined the possibility that different criteria may govern the admission of patients to the public and private sector. In order to consider this, it was decided to examine two geographically disparate Regional Secure Units and the one existing private medium secure hospital in order to compare the characteristics of patients admitted during the period 1989–92. This chapter focuses on the study of two RSUs, namely the Hutton Unit, Middlesbrough and the Norvic Clinic, Norwich and the following chapter will describe the study of Stockton Hall which is a medium secure private psychiatric hospital.

Before describing the first study, it is necessary to trace the development of the Regional Secure Unit to explain the place which such units occupy in the mental health system.

The Development of the Regional Secure Unit

Prior to the development of the Regional Secure Unit, the only psychiatric provision for the mentally ill was either the psychiatric ward of an NHS general hospital, or one of the Special Hospitals. The former had little or no security, the latter had maximum security. There was a complete absence of any middle ground in terms of psychiatric provision and so if any security at all was needed for a patient, the Special Hospitals would be called upon to provide this. Inevitably this meant that Special Hospitals had too many patients, many of whom did not require conditions of maximum security but who did require something more than could be offered by an NHS psychiatric ward. It also meant that some NHS wards contained patients whom psychiatrists were unwilling to consign to maximum security. As a result, the concept of the regional medium secure hospital originated in the 1957 report of the Royal Commission. This proposed that mentally ill patients who were particularly dangerous should be accommodated in hospitals with suitable facilities for their treatment and detention. This idea was floated by the (then) Ministry of Health and put to regional hospital boards in 1959. Two alternatives were originally suggested as ways of realising this. One idea was to introduce a secure psychiatric unit to every hospital. This was abandoned in favour of the idea of the Regional Secure Unit. These were to be freestanding specialist psychiatric hospitals based in different regions of the country where patients could be detained, near their homes, in conditions of medium security.

Initially, only the Northgate Clinic was built (now an adolescent unit) and in 1971 the Department of Health (which had replaced the Ministry of Health) reiterated that the plan to build regional secure units should proceed without further delay. In the same year, a working party was established under the chairmanship of Dr J.E. Glancy to review and make recommendations regarding the current and possible future need for secure provision. The Glancy Report (1974) recommended that regional health authorities should take the responsibility for providing secure units to deal with patients. This was, in part, reinforced a few months later by the Butler Committee Report on Mentally Ill Offenders (1975) which Gostin (1985, p. 33) cites as having stressed that:

> there [was] a 'yawning gap' between National Health Service Hospitals with no secure provision and the overcrowded Special Hospitals. The absence of any intermediate security, together with the development of treatment in open conditions in local hospitals has adverse effects on the Special Hospitals, the Criminal Justice System and the prisons.

The Butler Committee (1975) recommended that at least 2,000 secure places should be made available for patients requiring psychiatric care in conditions of medium security, for a period not usually longer than two years. The intention was that they would take the pressure off other facilities such as prisons and NHS hospitals which were either not equipped to deal with patients requiring medium secure psychiatric care, or in the case of the Special Hospitals, which had been overwhelmed with patients. The delay in going ahead with the opening of RSUs was due in part to a lack of funding, so it was suggested that regional health authorities should receive an allocation of money from central government to assist them in generating the necessary secure provision.

Although these recommendations were accepted by the government in 1974, progress was slow and further monies had to be promised as running costs before the units eventually got off the ground. It was not until 1984 that most regions had some sort of medium secure hospital unit or plans to provide permanent secure accommodation. In the North, the Hutton Unit at St Luke's Hospital, Middlesbrough was the first to be opened.

Bluglass stressed at this time that the greatest danger to these facilities was financial, and pre-empted the possibility that:

> [O]ther medical specialities will always be strong competitors for limited resources and it requires a firm commitment on the part of regional health authorities and central government to ensure the continued support that the units require (Gostin, 1985, p. 35).

In the light of this, the study seeks to address the respective contributions of the RSU and the private medium secure psychiatric hospital in terms of the service they provide to patients requiring their care. It aims to find out more about how patient access to such units comes about and whether there are any differences in the types of patient admitted, their source and the circumstances under which they come to be in secure psychiatric care. The motivation for any disparities found will then be discussed.

The Study

This chapter describes the study carried out at two Regional Secure Units. These were the Hutton Unit at St Luke's Hospital Middlesbrough and the Norvic Clinic in Norwich. Geographically disparate RSUs were chosen in order to allow for any regional variables which might have affected their admissions procedures. It was felt that this would provide a more fair and accurate comparison with the study done at Stockton Hall, York (the private psychiatric hospital the study of which is described in chapter 6).

The study comprised 84 patients admitted to the Hutton Unit and 93 patients admitted to the Norvic Clinic between 1989 and 1992. The data was collected from this period because it was the same time frame as data which had already been collected from Stockton Hall. Information came from patient files which contained psychiatric reports, court reports, medical notes and other information. A data collection sheet was used to collect the items needed for the study and all patients were number coded to protect their identities.

The sample comprised all patient files to which there was access in medical records, for the period 1989–92. Files not included in the sample were those not physically available. These were files belonging to some of the current patients who could have been admitted between 1989 and 1992, but whose file was currently on the ward or in the possession of the forensic psychiatrist. Data on the total number of patients admitted during this time was unfortunately not available to me. Whilst every effort was made to gain access to all files which may have been used in the study, the constraints of carrying out this type of fieldwork were many and varied.

It should also be noted that not all patient files consistently contained the same sort of data and collection of the relevant details required for the study was entirely dependent on the information contained in the medical files. In some cases therefore, data was not available and for the purposes of this study is recorded as such.

Before describing the study it is necessary to say that the reader may be disappointed by the small volume and lack of variety in the empirical work reported in the book. So is the writer. I came to Stockton Hall, the Hutton Unit and the Norvic Clinic well aware of the range of researchable topics. For instance, interviews suggested that the process of admission to Stockton Hall was much less bureaucratic than in RSUs, with admission decisions being made speedily, by staff operating alone rather than committee, and relatively fearlessly. To research this, a cohort of cases *considered* by Stockton Hall and the RSUs was necessary, with comparison of rejected as well as accepted cases. Exploring this possibility, it quickly became clear that the necessary data was not kept. A similar fate befell other approaches. It quickly became evident that patient surveys offered the only practicable way of beginning to gain insight into the processes at work. The reality of such surveys, with lengthy journeys to gather the data, the elusiveness of some files within the institution, and the suspicions of the research entertained by new management at Stockton Hall all conspired to change what should have been a modest piece of work into a mammoth task. Anyone similarly placed would have experienced similar problems. Perhaps one basic lesson is that empirical work is many times more time-intensive than one may imagine.

Results

Demographic Characteristics

In terms of age, Table 5.1 demonstrates that the largest group for both units fell within the 20–29 year age band. This was 33 (40 per cent) patients at the Hutton Unit and 37 (40 per cent) patients at the Norvic Clinic. This was closely followed by the 30–39 year age band in which there were 28 (33 per cent) at the Hutton and 30 (32 per cent) at the Norvic. There was also a fairly substantial number of patients whose age fell within the 40–49 year age band. This was 19 (22 per cent) at the Hutton and 19 (20 per cent) at the Norvic. Admission of patients either younger than 20 years or older than 50 years amounted to only 11 of the total joint cohort of patients admitted to both facilities during this time. No patients were admitted to the Hutton Unit under the age of 20 during this period and only six of that age to the Norvic Clinic. Similarly, only four patients over 50 years were admitted to the Hutton and one to the Norvic.

Table 5.1 Demographic characteristics

Age at admission	Hutton Unit		Norvic Clinic	
Under 20			6	(7%)
20 – 29	33	(40%)	37	(40%)
30 – 39	28	(33%)	30	(32%)
40 – 49	19	(22%)	19	(20%)
50 and over	4	(5%)	1	(1%)
Ethnic origin				
UK European	78	(94%)	85	(91%)
Caribbean			1	(1%)
Other European	1	(1%)	1	(1%)
African	2	(2%)	6	(7%)
Asian	2	(2%)		
No data	1	(1%)		
Gender				
Male	76	(91%)	79	(85%)
Female	8	(9%)	14	(15%)

Table 5.1 also shows the ethnic origin of the patients admitted to these two facilities. The highest proportion are Caucasian in origin. This amounts to 78 (94 per cent) of the total admissions to the Hutton and 85 (91 per cent) of the total admissions to the Norvic. The remaining 14 patients from both RSUs were of Caribbean, other European, African or Asian origin. For one patient, data on ethnic origin was not recorded.

In terms of gender mix, Table 5.1 also displays the predominance of male admissions to both facilities. 155 of the total of 177 admissions were male, the breakdown being 76 (91 per cent) male admissions to the Hutton, 79 (85 per cent) male admissions to the Norvic and eight (nine per cent) and 14 (15 per cent) female admissions to the Hutton and Norvic respectively.

Source of Admission

The location of all the patients immediately prior to their admission to these facilities was identified. Table 5.2 demonstrates that a significant number of admissions to both the Hutton and the Norvic came from other secure facilities. This was 62 (73 per cent) at the Hutton and 41 (44 per cent) at the Norvic. However, there was a more even spread of admissions from both secure and non-secure facilities to the Norvic Clinic which had 52 (56 per cent) patients admitted from non-secure facilities compared with the 22 (27 per cent) patients admitted from non-secure facilities to the Hutton Unit. The difference can be

Table 5.2   Source of admission

	Hutton Clinic		Norvic Clinic	
Secure facilities				
Prison	48	(57%)	31	(34%)
Regional Secure Units	1	(1%)	2	(2%)
Private psychiatric hospital				
Special hospital	11	(13%)	3	(3%)
Police cells	2	(2%)	5	(5%)
Secure juvenile accommodation				
Total	62	(73%)	41	(44%)
Non-secure facilities				
NHS non-secure wards	12	(15%)	6	(7%)
Community	10	(12%)	46	(49%)
Children's homes				
Total	22	(27%)	52	(56%)

explained by reference to the fact that the Hutton Unit took a greater proportion of referrals from prison and Special Hospitals than the Norvic Clinic, 48 (57 per cent) and 11 (13 per cent) patients respectively, whilst the Norvic took its greatest number of referrals from the community.

Table 5.2 demonstrates the substantial difference in referrals from the community between the Hutton Unit and the Norvic Clinic, showing this as only 10 (12 per cent) patients referred from the community to the Hutton Unit, but 46 (49 per cent) patients referred from the community to the Norvic Clinic.

An interesting feature of these admissions was that patients referred from other secure facilities were identified as being in need of care and treatment, whereas those referred from non-secure facilities were mainly admitted as a result of being identified as 'unmanageable' in that setting.

Authority for Detention

Table 5.3 summarises the authority for the detention of patients in both facilities. It demonstrates that the majority were detained in terms of the Mental Health Act 1983, Parts 2 and 3. A small proportion were classified as informal. This was two (two per cent) patients at the Hutton and 19 (21 per cent) patients at the Norvic. For a small number (less than five per cent in both facilities) there was no information regarding detaining orders in the files to which I had access and there was no alternative but to record this as such.

Of the 84 patients in the Hutton study, 15 (18 per cent) were detained in terms of the sections which form Part 2 of the Act. Of the 93 detained at the Norvic, 10 (11 per cent) were detained under Part 2. This part of the Act concerns civil detention where patients are admitted to hospital under section 2 for assessment or under section 3 which is the treatment order.

The remaining patients, who numbered 64 (75 per cent) at the Hutton and 60 (64 per cent) at the Norvic, were detained under Part 3 of the Act which concerns criminal proceedings or serving sentences. In these cases, the following number of patients were detained under the following sections.

Ten (12 per cent) patients at the Hutton and 31 (33 per cent) at the Norvic were detained under section 35 (admission to hospital for assessment); 6 (7 per cent) Hutton patients and 16 (17 per cent) Norvic patients detained under section 37 (the hospital order); 12 (14 per cent) Hutton patients and two (two per cent) Norvic patients were detained under section 37/41 (the hospital order with restriction); two (one per cent) Hutton and one (one per cent) Norvic patient detained under section 38 (the interim treatment order); seven (eight

Table 5.3   Authority for detention

			Hutton Unit		Norvic Clinic	
Formal patients	Part 2 MHA 1983	Section 2	4	(5%)	3	(3%)
		Section 3	11	(13%)	7	(8%)
	Part 3 MHA 1983	Section 35	10	(12%)	31	(33%)
		Section 37	6	(7%)	16	(17%)
		Section 37/41	12	(14%)	2	(2%)
		Section 38	2	(2%)	1	(1%)
		Section 47	7	(8%)	1	(1%)
		Section 47/49	7	(8%)	5	(6%)
		Section 48	12	(14%)	1	(1%)
		Section 48/49 C.P.I.	8	(10%)	3	(3%)
Total (formal patients)			79	(94%)	70	(75%)
Informal patients			2	(2%)	19	(21%)
No data			3	(4%)	4	(4%)
Total (informal patients)			2	(2%)	19	(21%)

per cent) Hutton and one (one per cent) Norvic patient was detained under section 47 (admission to hospital of sentenced prisoners); seven (eight per cent) Hutton and five (six per cent) Norvic patients were detained under section 47/49 (the transfer of remand prisoners to hospital); 12 (14 per cent) Hutton and one (one per cent) Norvic patient was detained under section 48 (admission to hospital of other prisoners, e.g. remand/immigration, etc.); and finally eight (10 per cent) Hutton and three (three per cent) Norvic patients were detained under section 48/49 (the transfer of a sentenced prisoner to hospital with restriction order).

Psychiatric Diagnosis

The primary psychiatric diagnosis was identified in 175 of the 177 admissions studied. In two cases, the files to which I had access did not record this information. These data are presented in Table 5.4 which illustrates the range of psychiatric diagnoses for the patients within this cohort.

At the Hutton Unit, these diagnoses were made in terms of DSMIIIR mental disorder classifications, but for the purposes of this study these have been translated into the more usual verbal descriptions of mental illnesses as these were the ones used both at the Norvic Clinic and at Stockton Hall and so are easier to compare.

Table 5.4 illustrates that the largest numbers of patients were diagnosed as suffering from schizophrenia, paranoid schizophrenia, personality disorder, manic depressive psychosis, mental impairment and mood disorder which included forms of clinical depression.

A diagnosis of schizophrenia was present in nine (11 per cent) of the Hutton admissions and 28 (30 per cent) of the Norvic admissions. The Hutton Unit also had 24 (29 per cent) patients diagnosed as paranoid schizophrenics whereas the Norvic had no patients detained with this diagnosis. A diagnosis of personality disorder was present in 17 (20 per cent) Hutton admissions and 20 (22 per cent) Norvic admissions. Eighteen (19 per cent) Norvic admissions were identified as suffering from manic depressive psychosis, compared to no patients with this diagnosis detained at the Hutton Unit.

Other significant diagnostic cohorts were paranoid state, drug induced psychosis and mental handicap or impairment, although these categories were not as prevalent as the former categories. Five (six per cent) Norvic patients were suffering from paranoid state compared to only one patient at the Hutton. Six (seven per cent) Hutton patients were diagnosed with drug induced psychosis compared to two patients at the Norvic and similarly seven (nine per cent) Hutton patients but only two Norvic patients were mentally handicapped or impaired.

Table 5.4   Psychiatric diagnosis

	Hutton Unit		Norvic Clinic	
Schizophrenia	9	(11%)	28	(30%)
Paranoid schizophrenia	24	(29%)		
Paranoid state	1	(1%)	5	(6%)
Personality disorder	17	(20%)	20	(22%)
Manic depressive psychosis			18	(19%)
Drug induced psychosis	6	(7%)	2	(2%)
Mood disorder/depression	16	(19%)	3	(3%)
Psychopath			3	(3%)
Organic state	1	(1%)	2	(2%)
Neurosis	1	(1%)	2	(2%)
Mental handicap/impariment	7	(9%)	2	(2%)
Schizo-affective disorder	1	(1%)		
Chronic alcoholism			1	(1%)
No mental illness diagnosed			6	(7%)
No data	1	(1%)	1	(1%)

In six (seven per cent) of the Norvic patients, no mental illness was present. All patients admitted to the Hutton Unit during the same period were found to have a recognisable mental illness. A few patients (one or two in each category) were found to be suffering from other psychiatric or organic illnesses such as neurosis, schizo-affective disorder, chronic alcoholism or organic state. Psychopathy was present in three (three per cent) Norvic patients but not found in any Hutton patients.

All admissions in the study were examined for a history of mental illness resulting in previous psychiatric hospitalisation. This was identified in 56 (67 per cent) Hutton patients and 55 (59 per cent) Norvic patients.

Criminal History

Table 5.5 illustrates that 58 (69 per cent) of the patients admitted to the Hutton Unit and 59 (64 per cent) of those admitted to the Norvic Clinic had a history of criminal convictions. The majority of these were property offences, arson or malicious damage and sexual or nonsexual violence. Relatively few patients had multiple convictions; 11 (13 per cent) at the Hutton Unit and 26 (28 per cent) at the Norvic Clinic. A large proportion had no recorded convictions. This accounted for 19 (23 per cent) Hutton patients and 30 (32 per cent) Norvic patients. In a small number of cases, this data was not recorded in the medical files of the patients.

Table 5.5   Criminal history

	Hutton Unit		Norvic Clinic	
None	19	(23%)	30	(32%)
Property offences	18	(21%)	14	(15%)
Arson/malicious damage	8	(10%)	6	(7%)
Manslaughter	1	(1%)		
Attempted murder	1	(1%)		
Murder	1	(1%)	1	(1%)
Sexual offences	4	(5%)	5	(5%)
Nonsexual violence	9	(11%)	7	(8%)
Property and sexual offences	1	(1%)		
Property and nonsexual offences	4	(5%)		
Multiple convictions	11	(13%)	26	(28%)
No data	7	(8%)	4	(4%)

Previous Institutional/Psychiatric Care

Table 5.6 illustrates the types of institutional and/or psychiatric care received by patients admitted during this time. In both cases, 10 patients had no previous institutional or psychiatric care recorded. Most patients had previously been detained in prison, Special Hospitals, other RSUs or National Health Service hospital wards. This comprised 10 (12 per cent) Hutton patients and 23 (24 per cent) Norvic patients previously detained in prison; nine (11 per cent) Hutton and five (six per cent) Norvic patients previously detained in Special Hospitals; three (four per cent) Hutton and 13 (14 per cent) Norvic patients previously detained in a Regional Secure Unit, and 22 (26 per cent) Hutton and 17 (18 per cent) Norvic patients previously in an NHS ward.

Table 5.6   Previous institutional/psychiatric care

	Hutton Unit		Norvic Clinic	
None	10	(12%)	10	(11%)
Prison	10	(12%)	23	(24%)
Special hospital	9	(11%)	5	(6%)
Regional Secure Unit	3	(4%)	13	(14%)
NHS ward	22	(26%)	17	(18%)
Special school	2	(2%)	2	(2%)
Private hospital			3	(3%)
Prison and RSU	2	(2%)	6	(7%)
Prison and special school	2	(2%)	2	(2%)
Prison and NHS ward	7	(9%)	5	(6%)
Prison, RSU and special hospital			1	(1%)
RSU and special school			2	(2%)
NHS and special hospital	4	(5%)		
RSU and special hospital	3	(4%)		
NHS and special school	2	(2%)		
Special hospital and special school	1	(1%)		
RSU and NHS			1	(1%)
Prison, RSU and special school			1	(1%)
Prison, RSU and special hospital	1	(1%)		
NHS, RSU and special hospital	1	(1%)		
RSU, special hospital and special school		1	(1%)	
Youth detention			1	(1%)
Adolescent unit			1	(1%)
No data	4	(5%)		

The remaining patients in both facilities had been detained in two or more facilities previously. Data was not available in four Hutton Unit patient files.

Discharge Details

The maximum observed length of stay of patients at the Hutton Unit during this time was 779 and for the Norvic Clinic it was 614 days. The mean length of stay was 149 days at the Hutton Unit and 115 days at the Norvic Clinic. Data were collected for all but one of the Norvic patients who may or may not have been discharged as there was very little information in the file.

Four patients continued to reside at the Hutton Unit at the time of the study and for 10 (12 per cent) patients no data was available.

The comments made therefore only apply to those patients for whom the details were recorded and available.

Table 5.7 illustrates the range of facilities to which the patients were discharged and their level of security. Of the Hutton Unit patients, 46 (55 per cent) were discharged to less secure facilities, three (three per cent) to facilities of the same level of security and 21 (24 per cent) to more secure settings. Of the Norvic patients, 41 (44 per cent) were discharged to less secure accommodation, six (six per cent) to accommodation of the same security and 45 (46 per cent) to more secure accommodation.

Table 5.7   Discharge details

		Hutton Unit		Norvic Clinic	
Less secure facilities	NHS wards	26	(31%)	24	(26%)
	Community	20	(24%)	17	(18%)
		46	(55%)	41	(44%)
Same level of security	RSU	2	(2%)	2	(2%)
	Private hospital			4	(4%)
	Special care unit	1	(1%)		
		3	(3%)	6	(7%)
More secure facilities	Prison	9	(11%)	40	(42%)
	Special hospital	12	(14%)	5	(6%)
		21	(25%)	45	(48%)
	No data	10	(12%)	1	(1%)
	Current patients	4	(4%)		

It would obviously have been difficult to say whether any of these results could be classed as significant without further analysis. For this reason the composite variables were broken down and compared in respect of the Hutton Unit and the Norvic Clinic and in Tables 5.8 to 5.13 the numbers in the cells represent observed and expected frequencies. It is possible from this data to test the results using the chi-square distribution. This measures the discrepancy existing between the observed and expected frequencies and if chi-square is greater than the critical value of chi-square the observed result is taken to be significant and the null hypothesis on which the expected frequencies have been determined can be rejected. The results of this testing was as follows.

Observed and Expected Frequencies

Demographic characteristics Table 5.8 illustrates that both the Hutton Unit and the Norvic Clinic admitted more male than female patients and more UK patients than any other. However, in terms of gender, the chi-square was 1.18 and in terms of ethnic origin it was 1.42. As the critical level for both of these results was 3.84 (1df) this means that these results are not significant.

Table 5.8   Demographic characteristics

Gender	Hutton Clinic		Norvic Clinic	
Male	76	(73.6)	79	(81.4)
Female	8	(10.4)	14	(11.6)
Ethnic origin	**Hutton Unit**		**Norvic Clinic**	
UK	78	(77.4)	85	(85.6)
Other	5	(6.2)	8	(6.8)

Source of admission Table 5.9 illustrates that more patients were admitted to the Hutton Unit from Special Hospitals than either a) were admitted from the same source to the Norvic Clinic or b) than might have been expected. The same appears to be true in respect of NHS referrals to the Hutton Unit. Also, there appears to be substantially more patients referred to the Norvic Clinic for care and treatment (where the referrals would have been made by prisons, courts or the police, etc.) than there were either to the Hutton Unit or than might have been expected from the results.

In this case the chi-square is 15.2 and the critical level is 15.1 (5df), so p< 0.01. The result is therefore reliable and there is a significant difference between the Hutton Unit and the Norvic Clinic in terms of the source of their patients.

Table 5.9   Source of admission

	Hutton Unit		Norvic Clinic	
Transfer RSU	1	(1.4)	2	(1.6)
Transfer special hospital	11	(6.6)	3	(7.4)
Transfer NHS	12	(8.5)	6	(9.5)
Community	4	(2.8)	2	(3.2)
Care and treatment	52	(62.6)	80	(69.4)
Other	4	(1.9)	0	(2.1)

Authority for detention Table 5.10 illustrates that in terms of s.35 which is admission to hospital for assessment, the Norvic Clinic had more patients than the Hutton Unit detained in terms of s.35. This is also a greater number than might have been expected as the observed frequency is 31 and the expected is 21.5.

Table 5.10   Authority for detention

MHA 1983	Hutton Unit		Norvic Clinic	
Section 3	11	(8.5)	7	(9.5)
Section 37	6	(10.4)	16	(11.6)
Section 37/41	12	(6.6)	2	(7.4)
Section 47	7	(3.8)	1	(4.2)
Section 47/49	7	(5.7)	5	(6.3)
Section 35	10	(19.5)	31	(21.6)
Section 38	2	(0.9)	1	(1.1)
Section 48	12	(6.2)	1	(6.8)
Section 48/49	8	(5.2)	3	(5.8)
Other	6	(11.9)	22	(13.1)

In terms of s.48 which is the admission to hospital of other prisoners (such as remand or immigration), the Hutton Unit had more s.48 patient than the Norvic Clinic and also more than might have been expected (observed 12, expected 6.5).

In terms of admissions under s.37, the hospital order and s.37/41 which is the hospital order with restrictions, the Norvic Clinic had more admissions under the former than the Hutton and the Hutton Clinic more under the latter than the Norvic Clinic.

Applying chi-square to the observed and expected frequencies the result is that chi-square is 51.81 (10df) and p< 0.001. The result is reliable and therefore it is possible to say that there is a significant difference in the authority for detention between the Hutton Unit and the Norvic Clinic and that the Hutton Unit were admitting more patients with restriction orders and other prisoners under s.48 than the Norvic Clinic.

Criminal history Table 5.11 demonstrates the observed and expected frequencies in respect of patients' criminal histories. It is regarded as usual to test for significance using chi-square at the five per cent level. Using this method for Table 5.11, the chi-square is 12.93 and the critical level (7df) is 14.1. The result at this level is therefore not significant. However, testing at the 10 per cent level it is possible to say that the result is significant as the critical level becomes 12.0 (7df) and therefore p< 0.1.

Table 5.11   Criminal history

	Hutton Unit		Norvic Clinic	
Property	18	(17.6)	14	(19.4)
Criminal damage	8	(6.6)	6	(7.4)
Manslaughter	1	(0.5)	0	(0.5)
Attempted murder	1	(0.5)	0	(0.5)
Murder	1	(0.9)	1	(1.1)
Sexual offences	4	(4.7)	5	(5.3)
Nonsexual violence	13	(9.5)	7	(10.5)
Multiple	11	(17.6)	26	(19.4)

This means that the Norvic Clinic admitted significantly more patients with multiple convictions than the Hutton Unit.

Previous institutional care Table 5.12 illustrates the observed and expected frequencies based on the numbers of patients who had previously been in other institutions during their lifetime. Here, the chi-square is 19.4 and the critical level 18.5 (4df), so p< 0.001. It is possible to say therefore that significantly more patients at the Norvic Clinic had previously been in prisons than those at the Hutton Unit and that more Hutton patients had previously been admitted to NHS facilities.

Table 5.12   Previous institutional care

	Hutton Clinic		Norvic Clinic	
Prison	22	(28)	37	(31)
Special school	8	(7.1)	7	(7.9)
RSU	11	(16.6)	24	(18.4)
Special hospital	19	(11.9)	6	(13.1)
NHS	37	(28.5)	23	(31.5)

Discharge details Table 5.13 demonstrates that the Hutton Unit moved fewer patients on to more secure facilities (relative to expectation) than did the Norvic Clinic. Here, the chi-square is 7.05 and the critical level is 5.99 (2df), so p<0.05. The result is again reliable so there is a significant difference between the Hutton Unit and the Norvic Clinic in the security level of the facilities their patients are discharged to and by inspection it appears to be the case that patients from the Norvic Clinic are discharged to facilities of higher security.

Table 5.13   Discharge details

Level of security	Hutton Unit		Norvic Clinic	
Lower	46	(37.6)	41	(49.4)
Same	3	(3.9)	6	(5.1)
Higher	21	(28.5)	45	(37.5)

Discussion

It was noted at the start of this chapter that the development of the Regional Secure Unit came about because of recommendations made in the Emery Report (1961), the Glancy Report (1974) and by the Butler Committee (1975).

The purpose of the Regional Secure Unit was to reduce the demand for beds currently being made on the Special Hospitals and to assist the prison population by reducing the numbers of seriously mentally ill prisoners.

It was widely accepted since the National Health Service Act 1977, that the Secretary of State was under a duty to provide psychiatric accommodation for those people deemed to require it and it was in the light of this that regional health authorities took responsibility (with government assistance) for providing it.

By the mid 1980s, most regions had some sort of medium secure hospital unit or plans to provide such, but from the outset, there has been a documented shortfall in the number of available beds. This has been most authoritatively reported by the Reed Committee Report (1992) and more recently by Watson (1994). As such, the provision of this type of care remains a salient feature on the health care landscape.

There have been a few similar studies into regional medium secure psychiatric provision carried out before such as those done by Higgins (1981), Gudjonsson and MacKeith (1983) and Treasaden (1985). However, none has provided a comparison with private medium secure care. Ultimately, this will be what this study intends to do and therefore it is pertinent and timely to review the respective populations of these two Regional Secure Units in order to provide a feasible comparison with the information which will be discussed in chapter 6.

In respect of demographic characteristics, the findings appear fairly unremarkable. It is usual for the population of a Regional Secure Unit to be in the main male, Caucasian and primarily within the age range 20 to 40 years.

In terms of the source of referrals, Table 5.2 illustrates that the Hutton Unit took its largest quota from secure facilities. In total this is true of 62 (73 per cent) patients, of whom the majority came from prison and a small number from Special Hospitals. In comparison, the Norvic Clinic took its largest number (52 (55 per cent)) of referrals from non-secure facilities, of which 46 (49 per cent) came from community sources. Having said this, the Norvic Clinic had a more even spread of referrals from either secure or non-secure facilities, and had 41 (43 per cent) patients in the secure facility category, 31 (33 per cent) of whom had been referred from prison.

Overall, Table 5.2 illustrates that whilst the Hutton Unit took a higher percentage of referrals from secure facilities and the Norvic Clinic a higher percentage from non-secure facilities, in terms of fulfilling the purpose for which Regional Secure Units were introduced, both were apparently doing this in that they admitted patients not only from the local community but also from NHS wards, prisons and occasionally the Special Hospitals. There appear to be slightly different emphases on sources of patients, but some regional variation is to be expected.

Table 5.3 demonstrates that both units took the majority of their patients on a formal basis under the Mental Health Act 1983. The Norvic Clinic had a higher proportion of informal patients than the Hutton Unit, 21 per cent as opposed to only two per cent of patients. However, this could be explained by the fact that Table 5.2 illustrated that the Norvic had a slightly higher community referral rate and this could account for higher informal patient numbers, most of whom would come from the local community.

In examining the psychiatric diagnoses displayed in Table 5.4, the most common are schizophrenia, personality disorder and mood disorder. These are fairly unremarkable findings which appear to be fairly characteristic of studies of Special Hospital and Regional Secure Unit populations (Coid, 1991).

Patient criminal histories demonstrate a wide range of offences, although quite a significant proportion in both units had no history of criminal conviction. Table 5.5 shows these figures as 19 (22 per cent) Hutton patients and 30 (32 per cent) Norvic patients.

In terms of previous institutional or psychiatric care, the study revealed a similar number of patients in both units with no such care recorded. This represents 12 per cent of the Hutton Unit patients and 11 per cent of the Norvic Clinic patients. Outside this category, most patients had received care in an NHS facility or had been in prison. The Norvic Clinic also had a significant number of patients who had received care previously in an RSU. Finally, in terms of their discharge, Table 5.7 shows that the majority of Hutton patients were discharged to less secure facilities. A very small percentage (three per cent) were transferred to facilities of the same level of security, whilst 21 (25 per cent) patients went either to prison or to a Special Hospital. However, it is not clear how this data might be different if it were not for the fact that these details for 10 patients had not been recorded in the files to which I had access.

The Norvic Clinic had a more even spread of discharges to either less or more secure facilities. Table 5.7 shows these figures as 41 (44 per cent) patients to less secure and 45 (48 per cent) patients to more secure facilities. A small number were transferred to facilities of the same security as the unit. These figures can be classed as slightly more complete than those of the Hutton Unit as only one patient file did not contain this information. Subsequent analysis demonstrated in Table 5.13, illustrates that the number of patients from the Hutton Unit who were discharged to facilities of a higher security was actually significantly less than those discharged to higher security facilities by the Norvic Clinic.

In terms of these findings, it appears (with a few exceptions) that the characteristics of patients admitted to the Hutton Unit and the Norvic Clinic are broadly similar in nature and although they do accept referrals from quite a wide range of sources, both secure and non-secure, and discharge their patients to facilities of slightly different levels of security, they do appear to be fulfilling the purpose for which they were introduced in terms of relieving pressure on prisons, Special Hospitals and the psychiatric wards of NHS hospitals. They are also providing a service to the community in which they are situated.

These findings will be compared with those from Stockton Hall, a private, medium secure hospital in chapter 7. The reason for reporting these separately is the fact that a Regional Secure Unit is one type of facility and a private psychiatric hospital such as Stockton Hall is another type. Although it has been demonstrated that both RSUs appear to perform some similar functions, they also differ in some respects and have different emphases. This chapter illustrates that awareness of such differences and lends itself to a further comparison in chapter 7.

The following chapter illustrates the same study carried out at Stockton Hall psychiatric hospital, York. This is a recently opened independent, medium secure facility, offering broadly the same provision as that offered by the public sector RSUs and I will seek to address any differences in the characteristics of patients admitted there between 1989 and 1992.

6 Access to Independent Psychiatric Care: A Study of Admissions to Stockton Hall Psychiatric Hospital 1989–92

Chapter 5 illustrated the characteristics of patients admitted to two Regional Secure Units between 1989 and 1992. It demonstrated that referrals to these two facilities were broadly similar in nature and that they appeared to be fulfilling the role for which they were intended in removing the seriously mentally ill from prisons, taking the pressure off NHS psychiatric wards and the Special Hospitals and providing medium secure psychiatric care at a regional level.

This chapter reports a corresponding study carried out at Stockton Hall Psychiatric Hospital which is an independent, medium secure facility.

To date there has been no research carried out in respect of the contribution being made by the private sector to psychiatric care. As long ago as 1975, the Butler Committee recognised that good research was essential for developing clinical practice and management of patients. More recently this has been underlined by the Reed Report (1992) which stressed that increased efforts should be made to disseminate existing reviews, courses and data and that any real gaps in information available should be identified and filled.

The purpose of this chapter is to help fill this gap by delineating the characteristics of patients admitted to Stockton Hall and at the same time to provide a useful comparison with the same study carried out in the public sector. It will provide information on the respective contributions of the public and private sector to medium secure psychiatric care and more specifically will address the issue of variations in access to these facilities and the possible motivations which might explain them.

The Study

Stockton Hall Psychiatric Hospital is owned by Partnerships in Care plc (previously the psychiatric division of AMI Healthcare plc). It accepts patients of either sex between the ages of 16 and 60 with any form of mental disorder, drug or alcohol dependence, or mental impairment. Referrals are considered from any part of the NHS, including the Special Hospitals and Regional Secure Units.

The concept of the private psychiatric hospital has received a mixed reaction. Amongst other things, Coid (1991) reports that it has been accused of catering for 'márket niches' such as eating disorders, impotence and stress reactions. At the same time the Reed Report (1992) stressed that the voluntary and independent sectors were making important contributions to meeting the special needs of mentally disordered offenders.

It has also been suggested (Mental Health Act Commission, 1989) that the development of private units offering secure and special care can be seen as a direct result of Health Authorities' lack of provision of suitable facilities. Now that private psychiatric provision is here, the critical question should not be whether such facilities should be run for profit, but whether they are providing a service which is effective and comparable to that of established, public sector medium secure hospitals or if there are any differences and if so, why. This study, like that carried out at the Hutton Unit and the Norvic Clinic seeks to address the issue of access to private psychiatric care and illustrate possible differences in patient characteristics.

The study examined a census population of Stockton Hall patients resident in December 1992, together with all admissions to Stockton Hall since it opened in September 1989. This comprised 142 admissions of 138 different patients, four patients having been readmitted during the period of study. Of the 142 admissions, 74 patients had been admitted to and discharged from Stockton Hall between February 1989 and December 1992. The remaining 68 patients were resident at Stockton Hall in February 1993. The information for the study came from patient files which contained psychiatric reports, court reports, medical notes and other information. A data collection sheet was used to gather the selected items needed for the study and all patients were number coded to protect their identities. As with the Hutton Unit and Norvic Clinic study, not all patient files consistently contained the same data and in some cases, data was not available and is recorded as such.

Results

Demographic Characteristics

Table 6.1 illustrates that the largest group of admissions, 75 cases (53 per cent) fell within the 20–29 year age band. This is followed closely by patients aged between 30–39 years, comprising 39 admissions (28 per cent). Admissions of patients either younger than 20 years or older than 39 years amounted, in total, to only 28 admissions (19 per cent). One hundred and thirteen (80 per cent) admissions were male and 29 (20 per cent) female.

In terms of ethnic origin, 120 (85 per cent) patients were Caucasian in origin, followed by 10 (seven per cent) patients of Caribbean origin, leaving the remaining 13 (nine per cent) patients being of African or Asian origin.

Table 6.1   Demographic characteristics

Age at admission	Stockton Hall	
Under 20	13	(9%)
20–29	75	(53%)
30–39	39	(28%)
40–49	12	(8%)
50 and over	3	(2%)
Ethnic origin		
UK European	119	(84%)
Caribbean	10	(7%)
Other European	1	(1%)
African	7	(5%)
Asian	5	(3%)
No data		
Gender		
Male	113	(80%)
Female	29	(20%)

Source of Admission

Table 6.2 demonstrates the location of patients in the period before admission to Stockton Hall. This was identified in 141 of the 142 admissions. Seventy-two patients were in some type of secure facility prior to their admission to Stockton Hall. This comprised 32 (23 per cent) admissions who were in prison, 13 (nine per cent) who were in Regional Secure Units, seven (five per cent) from another Partnerships in Care hospital and five admissions (three per cent) from a Special Hospital. There were also 12 (nine per cent) admissions who were classified as being admitted from police cells or custody, through Mental Health Act orders, having recently been at liberty in the community. A further three (two per cent) admissions were from secure juvenile accommodation.

Sixty-nine patients were categorised as not being in a secure facility before admission. These consisted of 50 (36 per cent) from non-secure National Health Service Wards, 18 (12 per cent) from the community and two (one per cent) from a children's home.

Table 6.2   Source of admission

		Stockton Hall	
Secure facilities			
	Prison	32	(23%)
	Regional Secure Units	13	(9%)
	Other private psychiatric hospital	7	(5%)
Total	Special hospital	5	(3%)
	Police cells	12	(9%)
Non-secure facilities	Secure juvenile accommodation	3	(2%)
		72	(51%)
Total			
	NHS ward	50	(36%)
	Community	18	(12%)
	Children's home	2	(1%)
		70	(49%)

Admissions were also examined to determine if referral had previously been made to a Regional Secure Unit or Special Hospital. 17 (12 per cent) of the cases referred to Stockton Hall were identified as having been referred to a Regional Secure Unit before a referral to Stockton Hall, with the patient having been rejected by the Regional Secure Unit. A further three (two per cent) patients were identified as having been referred to Special Hospitals for care and treatment, but rejected. It is possible that there were other patients who had previously been referred to a Regional Secure Unit or a Special Hospital, but I was unable to identify this from the information on file.

Authority for Detention

The authority for the detention of patients in terms of the Mental Health Act 1983 is summarised in Table 6.3. Twenty-two (16 per cent) were classified as informal patients. This included a small number of patients who had been admitted to Stockton Hall in terms of Probation Orders or (in the instance of juveniles) Secure Accommodation Orders.

Of the 120 formally detained patients, 64 were detained in terms of sections which form Part 3 of the Mental Health Act 1983 (patients concerned with criminal proceedings or serving sentences). Forty-seven (33 per cent) were detained in terms of section 37 (hospital orders). Of these 47 patients 15 also had a restriction order in effect, in terms of section 41 of the Mental Health Act. The remaining patients detained under sections from Part 3 of the Mental Health Act comprised; three (two per cent) admissions detained in terms of section 35 (admission to hospital for assessment), one patient admitted in terms of section 38 (interim treatment order), four (three per cent) patients detained in terms of section 47/49 (transfer of a remand prisoner to hospital), six (four per cent) patients detained in terms of section 48/49 (transfer of a sentenced prisoner to hospital) and three (two per cent) patients detained in terms of the Criminal Procedure (Insanity) Act 1964.

Fifty-six (39 per cent) patients were detained under Part 2 of the Mental Health Act 1983 (civil detention). All of these patients were detained under

Table 6.3   Authority for detention

			Stockton Hall	
	Part 2 MHA 1983	Section 2		
		Section 3	56	(39%)
		Section 35	3	(2%)
		Section 37	32	(22%)
Formal patients		Section 37/41	15	(11%)
	Part 3 MHA 1983	Section 38	1	(1%)
		Section 47		
		Section 47/49	4	(3%)
		Section 48		
		Section 48/49	6	(4%)
		C.P.I.	3	(2%)
Total (formal patients)			120	(84%)
Informal patients			22	(16%)
Total (informal patients)			22	(16%)

section 3, the treatment order. No patient was detained under section 2 (admission of a patient to hospital for assessment). Of the 120 admissions detained in terms of the Mental Health Act, 82 (58 per cent) were classified as suffering from mental illness, 26 (18 per cent) from mental impairment, seven (five per cent) from psychopathic disorder and five (three per cent) admissions were classified as suffering from severe mental impairment.

Psychiatric Diagnosis

The primary psychiatric diagnosis was identified on 116 of the 142 admissions. This shortfall was due to patient medical files not having been completed consistently in every case, and as such I had no alternative but to record this as missing data.

A diagnosis of schizophrenia was present in 48 (34 per cent) admissions and a diagnosis of paranoid state in a further two (one per cent). Nine (six per cent) admissions were diagnosed as suffering from affective or manic depressive psychosis. Nineteen (14 per cent) were suffering from psychopathic disorder. Mental impairment was a primary diagnosis in 29 (21 per cent) admissions and severe mental impairment in a further six (four per cent) admissions. The remaining three (two per cent) patients were diagnosed as suffering from organic conditions.

Table 6.4   Psychiatric diagnosis

	Stockton Hall	
Schizophrenia	38	(27%)
Paranoid schizophrenia	10	(7%)
Paranoic state	2	(1%)
Personality disorder		
Manic depressive psychosis	9	(6%)
Drug induced psychosis		
Mood disorder/depression		
Psychopathy	19	(14%)
Organic state	3	(2%)
Neurosis		
Mental handicap	35	(25%)
Schizo-affective disorder		
Chronic alcoholism		
No mental illness diagnoses		
No data	26	(18%)

Criminal History

Of the admissions to Stockton Hall, 91 (64 per cent) had a history of criminal convictions. These are summarised in Table 6.5 and are: 22 (15 per cent) admissions with a history of property offences; 20 (14 per cent) with offences of arson or malicious damage; 26 (18 per cent) admissions with a history of violent nonsexual offences; and 14 (10 per cent) admissions with a history of sexual offences. A further four (three per cent) admissions had a history of attempted murder and three (two per cent) admissions had a conviction for homicide. Two (one per cent) admissions were classified as having multiple convictions for more than one of the above categories of offence.

Table 6.5   Criminal history

	Stockton Hall	
None	46	(33%)
Property offences	23	(15%)
Arson/malicious damage	22	(14%)
Manslaughter		
Attempted murder	4	(3%)
Murder	3	(2%)
Sexual offences	14	(10%)
Nonsexual violence	26	(18%)
Property and sexual offences		
Property and nonsexual offences		
Multiple convictions	2	(1%)
No data	5	(4%)

Previous Institutional/Psychiatric Care

All the admissions were examined for a history of mental disorder, resulting in earlier psychiatric hospitalisation before their present period of psychiatric care. Such a history was identified in 72 (51 per cent) admissions.

Table 6.6 also illustrates that 42 (30 per cent) patients had previously been detained in prison, 21 (15 per cent) patients had attended approved or special schools and six (four per cent) patients had received no previous institutional or psychiatric care prior to being admitted to Stockton Hall.

Table 6.6   Previous institutional/psychiatric care

	Stockton Hall	
None	6	(4%)
Prison	42	(30%)
Special hospital	10	(7%)
Regional Secure Unit	6	(4%)
NHS ward	43	(30%)
Approved/special school	21	(15%)
Other private hospital	13	(9%)
No data	1	(1%)

Discharge Details

The average length of stay of patients discharged from Stockton Hall was calculated as being 256 days. This does not however, take into account patients who were resident at Stockton Hall at the time of the study. A number of these patients had been resident at Stockton Hall since the hospital opened. This means that the average length of stay, of all patients admitted to Stockton Hall can be taken as being significantly in excess of 256 days.

At the time of the study, 74 (52 per cent) patients had been discharged from Stockton Hall. Thirty-two patients (43 per cent of the total discharges) were transferred to non-medium secure NHS psychiatric wards, four patients

Table 6.7   Discharge details

		Stockton Hall	
Less secure facilities	NHS ward	32	(22%)
	Community	21	(15%)
Same level of security	RSU	14	(10%)
	Other private hospital	4	(3%)
	Special care unit	18	(13%)
More secure facilities	Prisons	1	(1%)
	Special hospital	2	(1%)
		3	(2%)
	No data		
	Current patients	68	(48%)

(five per cent of total discharges) were transferred to another Partnerships in Care hospital, 14 patients (19 per cent of total discharges) were transferred to Regional Secure Units, two patients (three per cent of total discharges) were transferred to Special Hospitals and one patient was transferred back to prison. Twenty-one patients (28 per cent of total discharges) were transferred from Stockton Hall into the community. This was most frequently into some form of sheltered hostel type accommodation.

Discussion

The development of medium secure psychiatric care is well documented in a variety of sources, for instance, the Emery Report (1961), the Glancy Report (1974), the Butler Report (1975) and most recently by Snowden (1985). The subsequent delay in providing the recommended number of medium secure beds is also well documented, (Treasaden (1985), Berry (1986)) and this was mentioned in chapter 5. The continuing lack of provision in medium secure psychiatric treatment is ongoing, as recently documented by the Reed Report (1992). The development of medium secure psychiatric provision within Partnerships in Care, as well as other independent operators (such as St Andrews Hospital, Northampton) can be seen as a private sector, market orientated response to a national shortage of medium secure beds, possibly in particular, relating to patients who require medium secure care on a protracted basis.

The only study of patients admitted to medium secure private psychiatric care has been that of Coid (1991). The study examined patients who were receiving care from five health districts in private hospitals and considered the reasons why the patients' needs had not been met by their parent hospitals. An examination of a total population of a medium secure, independent private psychiatric hospital has not previously been undertaken.

The literature regarding admission studies of patients to forensic institutions, with which these results may be compared is limited. Naismith and Coldwell (1990), together with Tennent et al. (1974) describe admissions to Special Hospitals. This is, however, not a comparable population as the studies relate to maximum security psychiatric care. There are only three studies of admissions to Regional Secure Units, all now rather dated, these being Higgins (1981), Gudjonsson and MacKeith (1983) and Treasaden (1985). Of these three studies, the most recent examines the largest population of patients admitted to four interim secure units and is the most useful. The study, however, demonstrates different patient characteristics in admissions to different secure units, which illustrates a further difficulty in making constructive comparisons in respect of the Stockton Hall admissions population. Having made these cautionary comments in respect of comparing the Stockton Hall admission population with much earlier studies of admissions to RSUs it is timely and beneficial to be able to compare this study with that carried out at the Hutton Unit and Norvic Clinics respectively and which was described in chapter 5. This comparison will be demonstrated in chapter 8.

In respect of the Stockton Hall admissions study, the following observations can be made.

In relation to the demographic characteristics, the findings are unremarkable, except for a larger percentage of the admissions to Stockton Hall being female than one might expect in a Regional Secure Unit. In common with Regional Secure Units, Stockton Hall accepted referrals from a wide range of sources, but does appear to be accepting more patients from National Health Service wards and from the community than any of the admission populations in other Regional Secure Unit studies. In examining the authority for detention, in respect of the Mental Health Act 1983, the largest group at Stockton Hall comprised patients detained in terms of section 37 (the hospital order). This also appears to be a characteristic of Regional Secure Unit populations. Stockton Hall admitted more patients detained in terms of section 3 (the treatment order) than appears to be demonstrated in Regional Secure Unit populations. Stockton Hall also had a relatively large number of informal patients, although this is not unique, there being a large number of informal patients at the Wessex Secure unit, when examined by Treasaden (1985).

In examining both the categories of mental illness in terms of the Mental Health Act 1983 and also the patient psychiatric diagnosis, there is a clear predominance of patients detained in terms of mental illness, the most common diagnosis being schizophrenia. This appears to be a characteristic of forensic psychiatric populations in general, similar findings being typical of examinations of populations of Special Hospitals as well as Regional Secure Unit studies. Stockton Hall did, however, appear to be admitting relatively few individuals suffering from psychopathic disorder. Patient criminal histories illustrated a wide range of offences, from the serious to the relatively minor, as appears to be the case in Regional Secure Unit populations. There did, however, appear to be an increased number of patients at Stockton Hall with no criminal history. Finally in terms of the discharge of patient, by far the largest number were discharged to facilities with a lesser degree of security, most commonly the community and NHS non-secure wards.

In addition to the characteristics of Stockton Hall patients already documented, other interesting features of the admission population were evident from patient files at the time of the data collection, which were not present in the files of the Hutton Unit and Norvic Clinic patients. A significant number of patients were identified in their medical files as being of exceptional difficulty in the management problems they posed. These difficulties related to repetitive, assaultive behaviour or repeated self injurious behaviour (such as self laceration). It was long term difficulties of this nature, together with resource implications, that appeared to provide the impetus for their health authority to fund a private psychiatric bed. It was also my impression that a significant number of Stockton Hall patients had received treatment there in excess of two years, although this was not demonstrated, as length of stay was only measured on patients discharged from Stockton Hall. If this observation is correct, it would reflect the absence of long term medium secure provision within the National Health Service, Regional Secure Units generally only being prepared to accept patients who require their services for two years or less.

Having established the general characteristics of Stockton Hall patients, and before embarking on a comparison with the study done at the Hutton Unit and the Norvic Clinic, it is pertinent in the light of the above comments, to investigate further those patients admitted to Stockton Hall who were recorded as having been admitted in circumstances relating to their exceptional difficulty. The reason for this is that such a cohort of patients was not identified in the files of the Hutton and Norvic patients and therefore this apparent disparity in access to these respective facilities merits further investigation. This will be discussed in the following chapter.

7 Access to Independent Psychiatric Care II: A Study of 59 Patients Identified as Unmanageable Prior to Admission to Stockton Hall Psychiatric Hospital 1989–92

Whilst undertaking data collection for the study described in chapter 6, it became evident from the medical files that a significant proportion of patients admitted to Stockton Hall were described within their files as having been 'unmanageable' in their parent district. This appeared to provide the impetus, for a number of reasons, for their subsequent referral to Stockton Hall. As the nature of this study was to focus on any disparities in access between public and private sector psychiatric provision, and as nothing similar had been evident in patient files at either the Hutton Unit or the Norvic Clinic, I decided to investigate this further. Data was subsequently collected regarding these patients to provide a useful insight into their characteristics, both medical and criminal and to address the question of how these patients came to find themselves not in secure psychiatric care within their own region, but in a private sector facility, often many miles away from their homes and families.

The Study

Additional study of the 142 patient files involved in the first Stockton Hall study described in chapter 6, revealed a cohort of 59 patients all of whom were recorded as having been admitted to Stockton Hall as a result of being identified as 'unmanageable' in their parent district. This data was collected on two occasions. The first was February 1993, when 36 patients had been discharged and 23 were still resident, and Tables 7.1–7.8 apply. The second period of data collection took place in February 1995. This covers the collection of data for the case study profiles of a representative sample of 20 of the 59 patients. How this sample was obtained will be described later. At the time of collection, all but four of the 59 patients in this study had been discharged. One patient was deceased. The reason for the two year time lapse was that (as indicated in an earlier chapter) access to the patient files at Stockton Hall had to be renegotiated and this took some time.

As before, the information gathered came from patient files which contained psychiatric reports, court and probation reports and medical notes as well as other information. A data collection sheet was completed for each patient and for reasons of confidentiality, all patients were number coded to protect their identities.

Results

Demographic Characteristics

The mean age of this cohort of 59 patients was 26 years. The gender mix was 45 (76 per cent) male and 14 (24 per cent) female. In terms of ethnic origin, 50 patients (85 per cent) were European, four (seven per cent) Asian, three (five per cent) Caribbean and the remaining two (three per cent), were African.

Source of Admission

Table 7.1 shows the location of all 59 patients immediately prior to their being admitted to Stockton Hall. The majority of these patients (54 (91 per cent)) were not in a secure facility before admission. The remaining five (nine per cent) patients had previously been resident in other private facilities or an acute psychiatric unit.

Of the patients categorised as not being admitted from a secure facility, 45 (75 per cent) were admitted from National Health Service wards, five (nine per cent) patients were admitted from the community, which in these cases indicates their own homes, two (three per cent) were from either a special school or a special needs boarding school, one (two per cent) was from a social services children's home, one (two per cent) from a hostel for the mentally handicapped and one (two per cent) from a community residential

Table 7.1   Source of admission

	Stockton Hall	
Secure facilities		
Other private hospital	4	(7%)
Acute psychiatric hospital	1	(2%)
Total	5	(9%)
Non-secure facilities		
NHS wards	45	(75%)
Community	4	(7%)
Special school	2	(3%)
Hostel for mentally handicapped	1	(2%)
Children's home	1	(2%)
Residential home	1	(2%)
Total	54	(91%)

home. Of the remaining four patients who were admitted from secure facilities, one (two per cent) was from an acute psychiatric unit and the other three (five per cent) were from other private psychiatric facilities. Of these, two patients were transferred from Kneesworth House and one from St Andrews Hospital.

All 59 patients were referred to Stockton Hall on the grounds of being classed as unmanageable in their current facility or location.

Behaviours Resulting in Admission to Private Care

Table 7.2 summarises the behaviours which were identified as resulting in patients being admitted to Stockton Hall between 1989 and December 1992. This table refers to the type of behaviour prevalent in the catchment area of the patient, whether this was in the community or in a local facility of some sort. Most of this behaviour was described in the patient files as purely 'unmanageable in current setting' and for the majority of patients (35 (59 per cent)), this term was used to describe generally disruptive or violent behaviour for which the parent facility/district did not have the resources to cope adequately. In a number of cases (24 (41 per cent)) however, the behaviour was more specifically described. Twelve patients (20 per cent) had been violent either to themselves or to others, four (seven per cent) posed an abscondence risk as they were not in secure facilities and needed to be. Three patients (five per cent) had assaulted staff in other facilities, three (five per cent) had refused to accept treatment, one (two per cent) had been setting fires and one (two per

Table 7.2 Behaviours resulting in admission to private care

	Stockton Hall	
Behaviour in parent district		
Unmanageable/disruptive behaviour	35	(59%)
Violence to self or others	12	(20%)
Abscondence risk	4	(7%)
Assaults on staff	3	(5%)
Refusal to accept treatment	3	(5%)
Fire-setting	1	(2%)
Sexually inappropriate behaviour	1	(2%)

cent) other had displayed sexually inappropriate behaviour on a consistent basis.

Of these patients, 17 had been referred to other facilities for care and treatment but had been rejected. In some cases, the Regional Secure Unit was reluctant to readmit patients who had previously posed problems. Others had been referred to Special Hospital but were rejected and for one patient there had been no bed available at Kneesworth House. It is possible that others within this cohort were similarly rejected by other facilities, but this information was not recorded in the files to which I had access.

Authority for Detention

Table 7.3 summarises the authority for the detention of patients under the Mental Health Act 1983. A small proportion of these (12 (20 per cent)) had been admitted either informally or under the terms of a secure accommodation order. One patient only was detained under s.2 which regulates the admission of patients to hospital for assessment. The majority (35 (59 per cent)), were detained under s.3 Mental Health Act which is the treatment order, whilst seven (12 per cent) were detained under s.37 (the hospital order), three (five per cent) under s.37/41 (hospital order with restriction order) and one patient in terms of the Criminal Procedure (Insanity) Act 1964.

Psychiatric Diagnosis

All 59 patients had an identified psychiatric diagnosis. A summary of this appears as Table 7.4.

The majority of the sample had a diagnosis of mental illness or

Table 7:3   Authority for detention

			Stockton Hall	
Formal patients (MHA 1983)	Part 2 MHA 1983	Section 2	1	(2%)
		Section 3	35	(59%)
	Part 3 MHA 1983	Section 37	7	(12%)
		Section 37/41	3	(5%)
		C.P.I.	1	(2%)
Total			47	(80%)
Others	Secure accommodation order		8	(14%)
	Informal		4	(6%)
Total			12	(20%)

Table 7.4   Psychiatric diagnosis

	Stockton Hall	
Mental illness/psychopathy	25	(43%)
Schizophrenia	19	(32%)
Mental impairment	9	(15%)
Personality disorder	4	(7%)
Brain damage/mental handicap	2	(3%)

psychopathy. This group comprised 25 patients (43 per cent of the sample). A further 19 (32 per cent) were diagnosed schizophrenic, whilst nine (15 per cent) were diagnosed as suffering from mental impairment. Four (7 per cent) patients had personality disorders and the remaining two (three per cent) were suffering from organic conditions such as brain damage or mental handicap. A history of previous mental disorder was found to be present in 53 (90 per cent) of the 59 cases studied.

Previous Psychiatric Care

Table 7.5 illustrates that 40 (68 per cent) of the patients admitted had already had previous psychiatric care in National Health Service wards. These figures are independent of those which outline the patients' source of admission immediately prior to Stockton Hall. Five patients (eight per cent) had previously been in both an NHS facility and a private facility, whilst one patient (two per cent) had previously been admitted to both an NHS facility and a Regional Secure Unit. Of the remaining patients, four (six per cent) had

Table 7.5   Previous psychiatric care

		Stockton Hall	
Non-secure facilities	NHS wards	40	(68%)
Secure facilities	Other private hospital	4	(6%)
	Special hospital	1	(2%)
	Children's psychiatric unit	1	(2%)
	Acute psychiatric hospital	1	(2%)
	NHS and other private hospital	5	(8%)
	NHS and RSU	1	(2%)
Other	No previous care	5	(8%)
	No data	1	(2%)

previously been admitted to another private hospital, one to a Special Hospital, one to an acute psychiatric unit and five (eight per cent) had received no psychiatric care. In one case there was no information available within the patient file.

Previous Institutional Care

The sample of admissions was also examined for previous institutional care, other than that coming within the ambit of psychiatric care.

Table 7.6 summarises the data, although this posed some problems because this type of information appeared not to be recorded as a general rule within the files to which I had access. This resulted in the fact that for 16 patients (27 per cent) I was unable to determine any previous institutional care. However, Table 7:.6 does show that in 29 cases (49 per cent) there was evidence of this

Table 7.6   Previous institutional care

	Stockton Hall	
None	14	(24%)
Prison	9	(15%)
Children's home/approved school	7	(12%)
Hostel/residential home	6	(10%)
Special school	4	(7%)
Adolescent unit	2	(3%)
Head injury/rehabilitation centre	1	(2%)
No data	16	(27%)

type of care. Nine (15 per cent) patients had previously experienced the penal system, seven (12 per cent) had been in a children's home or approved school, six (10 per cent) had been in a hostel or residential home, four (seven per cent) had been in a special school or special needs boarding school, two (three per cent) in an adolescent unit and 1 in a head injury rehabilitation centre. Fourteen patients (24 per cent) had no previous institutional care of this type.

Criminal History

Table 7.7 illustrates criminal history. Twenty-seven patients (46 per cent) had a history of criminal convictions, whilst 29 (49 per cent) had no previous criminal history. Those with a criminal history can be categorised as eight (14 per cent) with a history of arson/malicious damage, six (10 per cent) with a history of property offences, seven (12 per cent) with a history of nonsexual violence, four (seven per cent) with a history of sexual violence and two (three per cent) with a history of attempted murder. For three of the patients there was no information of this type within the medical files to which I had access. It is likely that, in spite of these results, some patients would have had a more varied criminal career but discrepancies in how personal details had been recorded in patient files was a major problem resulting in a lack of mixed records.

Table 7.7   Criminal history

	Stockton Hall	
None	29	(49%)
Arson/malicious damage	8	(14%)
Property offences	6	(10%)
Nonsexual violence	7	(12%)
Sexual offences	4	(7%)
Attempted murder	2	(2%)
No data	3	(5%)

Discharge Details

At the time of the study, 36 of the 59 patients had already been discharged from Stockton Hall, whilst the remaining 23 were still resident.

For the 36 discharges, the mean length of stay was 201 days. Table 7.8 summarises these details which can be categorised in the following way.

Thirteen (36 per cent) of the patients discharged returned to their regional NHS wards, 13 (36 per cent) returned to the community (here this indicates a discharge to the care of family or friends), and five (13 per cent) patients were transferred to another, private hospital. Of these, two patients went to St Andrews Hospital, Northampton, one to the adolescent unit at Langton House, Dorset and the remaining two were transferred to Kneesworth House hospital, Cambridge. Of the remaining five patients, one was transferred to prison, one to an acute psychiatric facility, one to a home for the mentally handicapped, one to a crisis intervention centre and one to the care of Sense in the Midlands.

In terms of the level of security at discharge, the preceding categories indicate that 28 (78 per cent) of the patients discharged at the time of the study went to less secure accommodation or facilities than Stockton Hall. Seven (19 per cent) patients were transferred to a location of the same level of security and only one patient was transferred to a more secure environment.

This means that Stockton Hall were able to discharge the majority of their patients to far less secure settings.

Table 7.8   Discharge details

		Stockton Hall *Patients discharged*	
Less secure facilities	NHS wards	13	(36%)
	Community	13	(36%)
	Crisis intervention centre	1	(3%)
	Sense	1	(3%)
		28	(78%)
Same level of security	Other private hospital	5	(13%)
	Acute psychiatric facility	1	(3%)
	Home for the mentally handicapped	1	(3%)
		7	(19%)
More secure	Prison	1	(3%)
Current patients		23	

Case Studies

Having initially discussed the overall characteristics of this cohort of 59 'unmanageable' patients, I decided to place greater focus on a random sample in terms of their life history and criminal careers, as far as the information to which I had access would allow. In their study of hospital order patients,

Gibbens and Robertson (1983, p. 362) emphasised the importance of studying these issues when they said, '[p]sychiatrists have long been aware of the importance of studying the life history of mentally ill patients'.

In the same way, with the recent advent of private psychiatric treatment for the mentally ill, little or nothing is actually known about the circumstances in which these patients are admitted to a private hospital. Having identified the not insignificant number of patients defined by other facilities as 'unmanageable' before admission to Stockton Hall, it appeared logical to address in more detail the circumstances which led to their admission and the reasons why they were classified unmanageable elsewhere. This helps to explain the motivation behind the willingness of Stockton Hall to admit those patients often defined as long-term difficult to manage and the disparity in access between Stockton Hall and the two Regional Secure Units in the study, for whom there were no patients recorded as being admitted for these reasons.

Method

A representative sample from the initial cohort of 59 patients was taken. This comprised 20 patients in total, of which 10 had been admitted from regional NHS facilities and 10 others who had been admitted from alternative sources which included the community, children's homes, special schools and other private hospitals. Of these, 14 were male and six female.

This sample appeared to be the most fair and representative of the cohort, as the study had shown that although most of the original 59 patients had been admitted from NHS facilities, there was also a significant number from other sources. A representative sample was therefore taken from each.

A further factor was the number of case studies to be profiled. Whilst it would theoretically have been possible to give an account of all 59 patients involved, this would probably have become an extremely tedious piece of literature to read. I felt under the circumstances that the sample of 20 would therefore be sufficient to illustrate any frequent admission characteristics.

The samples taken from each source were chosen randomly. The number codes given to each patient were written on slips of paper and divided into two piles, one whose source were NHS wards and the others. My (then) five-year-old daughter picked 10 slips of paper from each pile and these were the patients chosen for the study.

As far as the medical records to which I had access would allow, data was collected on the family histories of the patients, their psychiatric condition and diagnosis, any details regarding their criminal history and the circumstances, in as much detail as possible, regarding their admission to Stockton Hall Hospital. The patients had all been admitted between 1989 and 1992 and by February 1995, when this portion of the data was collected, all but four had been discharged. One patient was deceased. For the purposes of confidentiality, all patients retained their original number coding and are referred to throughout by this number. The case studies outlined first are those for whom the source of admission was NHS wards within their parent districts.

Case Study 1: Patient 49

This 51-year-old female patient had been admitted to Stockton Hall from her parent district NHS hospital under s.3 Mental Health Act 1983 in 1990.

Her parents were no longer alive but a history of mental illness on the mother's side was recorded. The patient had been born at home and had suffered convulsions from the age of four days. As a result, she did not develop properly as an infant and had not talked until the age of four years. Her vocabulary was severely limited and her IQ had been assessed at 38.

It was recorded that patient 49 had always been difficult to manage at home and at the age of eight, having been deemed incapable of school education, she was hospitalised. The diagnosis was primarily severe mental impairment and explosive personality. From approximately the age of 15 the patient was noted to be extremely difficult in terms of management, with a propensity for attacking staff and other patients.

At the age of 28, patient 49 was transferred to Rampton, a maximum security Special Hospital, where she was described as 'disturbed and violent', was frequently secluded and given to self-abuse. Until 1980, patient 49 was nursed in what is known at Rampton as 'Main Ward Block' which is for the more severely disturbed patients. She was then moved to a section called 'The Villa' which is for less disturbed patients. By 1981 the staff at Rampton felt that patient 49 no longer needed to be housed in conditions of maximum security and she was transferred to an NHS psychiatric ward in April 1982.

In this facility, patient 49 was described carrying out self-abuse and being a compulsive tea-drinker. In December 1986 she suffered a grand mal fit, although no previous epileptic phenomena had been present. She continued with frequent violent outbursts and also began experiencing auditory hallucinations. As a result, a diagnosis of schizophrenia was made. Nonetheless, arrangements were made for patient 49 to be discharged to a hostel in the community which proved unsuccessful due to her difficult and violent behaviour.

In December 1988, patient 49 was readmitted to an NHS psychiatric ward where she remained aggressive and disturbed and had to be secluded on many occasions. Her behaviour was deemed so unmanageable that staff felt she required a more suitable, secure hospital placement. Although this patient's parent district was London, a transfer was made to Stockton Hall in order to stabilise her condition with a view to the possibility that she might eventually return to her home area where she had a brother.

Patient 49 spent 844 days at Stockton Hall and was discharged to a nursing home in the South which provided less secure accommodation. As a result of spending the majority of her life in an institutionalised environment, she had no official criminal career.

Case Study 2: Patient 51

Patient 51 was a 28-year-old male who was admitted in 1992 to Stockton Hall from an NHS psychiatric ward under s.3 Mental Health Act 1983, having had a history of psychotic episodes and hypomania.

It was recorded that the patient's mother had schizophrenia and had been hospitalised on many occasions. The patient's father died in 1972 from cancer. Patient 51 was described as being 'pushed from pillar to post' as a child and had been looked after by an aunt and other relatives. He had attended normal primary school and the first year of junior school, but after his father's death had been placed in a children's home. He subsequently attended an education centre for children with behavioural problems until he was 16. During this time there had been a number of problems such as absconding, fighting, excessive drinking and glue-sniffing.

At the age of 16, the patient found employment in a local butcher's shop but left after breaking his arm. He then worked for a short time as a pest controller and a road sweeper, but had his first 'breakdown' in 1985.

It was recorded that patient 51 had been involved in criminal activities which appeared to be connected, in part at least, to the misuse of illegal drugs such as cannabis and LSD. He had been involved in theft, criminal damage, assault and threatening behaviour and had been in prison.

The patient had first been admitted to a an NHS psychiatric ward in 1985, following an arrest by the police. He was diagnosed as schizophrenic and was noted to be suffering from persecutory delusions and manic episodes. He was described as having 'smashed the place up' on a number of occasions and was frequently threatening to staff and other patients. He consistently ignored all medical advice and after throwing a fire extinguisher through a glass door was forcibly removed by the police and discharged from the hospital.

In 1989 patient 51 had five admissions to two different NHS psychiatric wards and one admission to Kneesworth House under s.3 Mental Health Act 1983. It was recorded that he made progress at Kneesworth and as a result was transferred back to his local NHS ward. He was then described as becoming 'totally unmanageable in an open ward situation'. The NHS facility refused to readmit him whereupon he was admitted to Stockton Hall.

Patient 51 spent 169 days at Stockton Hall. He was recorded as having responded to treatment and as a result was able to return to the NHS psychiatric ward in his parent district.

Case Study 3: Patient 59

Patient 59 was a 16-year-old admitted under a secure accommodation order from a National Health Service adolescent unit in 1989. He had been born four weeks premature, weighing 4lbs 5oz and had many periods in care during his early life due to his parents' ill health. He was described as an 'angry child' and as having few friends.

Patient 59 was first seen by an educational psychiatrist in 1980, in connection with his slow progress at school. Testing at this time showed him to be of limited intelligence and he was recommended for a Special Unit at Junior School. Whilst there, he was described as having behavioural problems which led to him being excluded twice.

At the age of 13, medical records describe the patient as 'abusive, insulting, prone to shoplifting and an abscondence risk'. He perpetrated violent attacks in school on both staff and other pupils which led to his transfer to a Children's Centre. He appeared to improve but began setting fires in 1987.

The patient's mother had suffered from chronic mental illness and after her death in 1985, patient 59 had suffered from unresolved grief. As a result he was considered suitable for inpatient treatment at his local Adolescent Unit. Unfortunately he proved to be totally unmanageable because of his persistent fire-raising and violence.

He was admitted to Stockton Hall in 1989 where he was diagnosed as suffering from an unsocialised conduct disorder. He spent 273 days at Stockton Hall before being discharged to a hostel in the community.

Case Study 4: Patient 64

Patient 64 was a 20-year-old male admitted to Stockton Hall in 1992 under s.3 MHA 1983 from his local National Health Service psychiatric ward.

The patient had been diagnosed as a schizophrenic at the age of 18. He had displayed this by becoming socially withdrawn and almost totally preoccupied with his own facial appearance. He was recorded as having a fairly normal childhood, although his parents had divorced when he was relatively young. It was also recorded that he heard voices and experienced bizarre delusions.

The patient's condition improved slightly on admission to his local hospital but after being discharged, he discontinued his medication and had to be readmitted. This became the pattern of events and when not on medication, patient 59 was extremely violent to staff in the hospital and to his own family. It was thought likely that he was abusing illicit drugs and his condition continued to deteriorate. He began assaulting staff and eventually assaulted his mother and then threw himself out of a window whilst on a visit home. As a result, his local hospital felt that no further progress would be made unless he was sectioned and the patient was admitted to Stockton Hall in 1992.

After an initial stay of 28 days, during which some progress was recorded, the patient was transferred back to his local hospital but had to be readmitted to Stockton Hall due to his continued and persistent unmanageability. Again some progress was made and the patient began to go home for short visits. Unfortunately, it was whilst he was on one such visit that patient 64 committed suicide by throwing himself under a train after arguing with his parents. He is one of two patients who have committed suicide at Stockton Hall since the hospital opened in 1989. The other suicide was committed on the premises.

Case Study 5: Patient 68

In comparison with the majority of the patients admitted to Stockton Hall, patient 68 presents an unusual profile in that he originates from a professional background, his father being a solicitor and his mother a lecturer. Patient 68 was a 20-year-old male admitted under s.3 MHA 1983 from his local NHS psychiatric ward in 1991. The patient had an older, adopted brother and a younger sister who suffered from a depressive illness and had a tendency to self-harm if under stress.

According to his parents, the patient started having problems at the age of 16 and they had wondered if this was connected with drug abuse. He had passed nine GCSEs and one A level, but left school to get a job and a flat. He admitted that during this time he was involved in taking and selling illegal drugs.

Some time later whilst on holiday in France, the patient became rather ill and had to be brought home by his brother. He began threatening his family and wrecked the house. His mother became very frightened of him and as a result he was admitted to the psychiatric ward of his local hospital. Later he was sectioned because he refused treatment.

Psychiatric assessment showed that patient 68 appeared to be psychotic as a result of drug abuse. It was also thought possible that he could be schizophrenic. After initial treatment, he was allowed home but the situation regarding his violence and unmanageability did not improve. At the suggestion of being returned to hospital, he took several knives from the kitchen and said that if the police came to take him back, he would attack them. He then began throwing the knives into his parent's lounge carpet. The psychiatric ward of the patient's local hospital did not want to readmit him and so he was transferred to Stockton Hall in November 1991. He remained there for 51 days and was then transferred back to his local NHS psychiatric ward.

Case Study 6: Patient 69

Patient 69 was a 25-year-old male admitted to Stockton Hall as a recall patient under s.3 MHA 1983 in 1992. He was admitted from his local NHS psychiatric ward.

This patient had been born at home as a breech delivery and was later diagnosed as having brain damage. He was transferred to a special care baby unit and for some time was paralysed down the right side. He presented with enormous feeding problems and was given a very poor prognosis at the time.

At the age of two, the patient began to display destructive behaviour. He later attended a local school for the educationally subnormal but had to leave at the age of eight because of his disruptive behaviour. He was moved to a special school which he attended until the age of 15.

At the special school unsuccessful attempts were made to teach the patient to read and write but his disruptive and violent behaviour made this impossible. He continued to destroy things and at home, threatened his parents. It was recorded that his language and behaviour centred around his own sexual fantasies involving his sisters and other women.

At the age of 16, the patient was moved to his local NHS psychiatric ward where he continued to be prone to destructive and violent outbursts. As a result he was admitted to Stockton Hall in 1991. After making some progress, he was discharged to his local NHS psychiatric ward but absconded. He returned to his parents' home, causing damage to their house and a number of cars. He was readmitted to Stockton Hall where he remained for 108 days and then was discharged to the care of his family.

Case Study 7: Patient 73

Patient 73 was a 17-year-old male admitted to Stockton Hall from the adolescent unit of his local NHS hospital under a secure accommodation order. He had a history of aggressive behaviour including assault and wounding. It was also recorded that he had extremely violent feelings towards women.

The patient's mother was recorded as being disturbed and having limited intelligence, with a psychiatric record. He also had a foster mother and a half-brother in his early 20s who was serving a life sentence for the murder of a young woman.

At the age of five, the patient had been put on the non-accidental injury register. He had attended normal schools until the age of eleven. He was then taken into care at his mother's request because of his violent and aggressive behaviour and attended a residential school for boys with learning difficulties.

In 1988 a full care order was made and he was placed with foster parents. His own mother objected to this and took him from the care of the foster parents to live with her in a hostel where they remained until 1990. He was then arrested for robbery and wounding and spent five months in a secure unit. He was then moved to an adolescent unit after making threats to women with a knife. Soon after this transfer, the resident adolescent psychiatrist sought the back-up of Stockton Hall because of this patient's extreme violence and abrupt mood swings. There were also fears concerning his ability to harbour resentment towards the nurses involved in his care, whom he often said he would 'like to repay'. He was recorded as showing no remorse after his frequent violent outbursts.

As a result, the patient was transferred to Stockton Hall. He was diagnosed as having an antisocial personality disorder which was probably due to his disturbed background and the lack of emotional stability in his formative years. Stockton Hall agreed to take him because of the extreme management difficulties he posed in his parent facility and proposed to settle him in order that he might eventually be found another well-supervised environment.

Patient 73 spent 56 days at Stockton Hall before being transferred to St Andrews Hospital, Northampton.

Case Study 8: Patient 79

Patient 79 was a 24-year-old female admitted under s.3 MHA 1983 from her local NHS psychiatric ward. She had a history of mental illness going back to the age of 11 and had presented a severe management problem for her local hospital. She was recorded as suffering from persecutory auditory hallucinations, was unable to control her aggressive behaviour and was abusive, incontinent and an absconscion risk.

The patient had apparently had a fairly normal childhood, but from the age of 12 displayed severe temper tantrums and began truanting from school. She left school at the age of 16 and completed a youth training scheme but was unable to find employment after this. She then became increasingly withdrawn until she stopped going out of the house altogether. She began to self-abuse and on one occasion used an electric drill. She attacked her parents and damaged the house and was then admitted to hospital.

Whilst in the psychiatric ward of her local hospital she accused her father of abusing her but later withdrew these allegations. She was moved briefly to a hostel, but this proved unsuccessful because she assaulted another resident with a knife and slashed her own wrists with a bread knife. She was readmitted to the psychiatric ward of the local hospital but assaulted the staff and then absconded in her nightdress. They were unable to cope with this sort of behaviour so she was transferred to Stockton Hall in 1992.

At the time of the study patient 79 was described as very disturbed and had not been discharged.

Case Study 9: Patient 92

Patient 92 was a 34-year-old female admitted from the psychiatric ward of her local NHS hospital under s.3 MHA 1983 in 1991. She was diagnosed as suffering from schizo-affective disorder.

Unfortunately there was very little information in this patient's files and I had no access to any other information. She had been known to her local hospital since 1983 and was recorded as living with her mother who had very little insight into her daughter's condition, describing her as 'not feeling well'. It was recorded that she thought she was being sent messages through the television set and had described seeing faces at the foot of her bed. She was prone to injuring herself and had swallowed lighted cigarettes, burned herself and had tried to drown herself in the bath. Her local hospital had tried a variety of treatments but felt that none of them had an appreciable effect.

They were unwilling to detain the patient any longer so she was transferred to Stockton Hall in 1991.

Case Study 10: Patient 99

The final patient in the cohort admitted from regional NHS psychiatric wards was patient 99 who was admitted under s.37/41 MHA 1983, in 1990.

This patient was a 47-year-old male who had suffered from paranoid schizophrenia since 1962 and had frequent admission to hospital. Details of this cannot be discussed in full because the medical notes for the years in question were not made available to me.

Between 1973 and 1981 patient 99 had been detained in Broadmoor Special Hospital where he was described as 'reasonably settled'. As a result he was transferred to a less secure hospital but his condition deteriorated. He began to abscond with frequency, on one occasion hitting a police officer over the head with a piece of scrap metal. He was arrested, convicted and sentenced for this offence. On his release from prison, his hospital and restriction orders were still in effect but his local hospitals were unwilling to admit him. He was therefore admitted to Stockton Hall.

At the time of the study, patient 99 was still resident at Stockton Hall. It was recorded that although he was no longer felt to be dangerous within certain confines, he would have difficulty living independently and that he acknowledged this. Attempts were being made to transfer him to the care of another hospital as a first step towards reintegrating him into the community

Case studies 11 to 20, which are now discussed, involve those patients whose source of admission to Stockton Hall was a source other than a National Health Service psychiatric ward.

Case Study 11: Patient 11

Patient 11 was a 28-year-old male admitted to Stockton Hall under s.3 MHA 1983 from his parent's home where he had been on a home visit from Kneesworth Hospital. The patient was the eldest of three children and had been born prematurely, weighing only 2lb 5oz. He was described as being slow to attain normal developmental milestones and left school at the age of 16, barely able to read or write.

The patient first began to show signs of mental disorder in 1984 when he became argumentative and aggressive towards his family. Shortly after this he was arrested by the police for damaging cars and was admitted to the psychiatric ward of his local hospital under s.136 MHA 1983. He was transferred to Kneesworth House Hospital in 1988, but discharged himself and continued to attend his local hospital as a psychiatric outpatient. Later in the same year he discontinued his medication and had to be readmitted to Kneesworth House.

During this time it was recorded that the patient was extremely aggressive and consistently displayed inappropriate sexual behaviour. On one occasion he had attempted to strangle his mother saying after that he thought she was the cat. The patient often exposed himself and was threatening towards his siblings. Psychiatric assessment described him as 'clearly psychotic' thinking himself to be the 'prophet of God'. He also maintained that people on the television set instructed him to do certain things and that he could control the weather. He was diagnosed schizophrenic and his medical records underlined the need for continued medication.

After being discharged from Kneesworth House, the patient moved into shared accommodation. This was not a success because he attacked the other occupants and at this point his local hospital said it was not prepared to readmit him because of the severe problems of management that he posed. As a result he was admitted from the community to Stockton Hall where he remained for 91 days. He was discharged into the care of his family.

Case Study 12: Patient 14

Patient 14 was a 23-year-old male admitted to Stockton Hall initially on an informal basis by his local Social Services department. This informal detention was subsequently changed to a s.3 detention under the terms of the MHA 1983.

This patient had been born with a condition called plagiocephaly (a closed skull) and as a result his development had been very slow. He was diagnosed at Great Ormond Street Hospital as mentally handicapped and had attended a school for children with learning difficulties. During this time he had lived with his family in a large house.

After the patient's father and grandfather died, the patient became much more difficult. His local Social Services department was informed of the situation in 1981 as a result of the patient perpetrating temper tantrums and threatening behaviour against his family and neighbours. After leaving school in 1987, plans were made for the patient to live independently. To prepare for this, he attended an independence training unit but began setting fires. As a result, no local facility would accept him so he was admitted to Stockton Hall at the request of the Social Services, for assessment.

The patient was diagnosed as mentally handicapped and remained at Stockton Hall for 468 days. He was discharged to a hostel in the community.

Case Study 13: Patient 27

Patient 27 was a 16-year-old male admitted to Stockton Hall under a secure accommodation order in 1991. He had been resident at a special needs boarding school from which he had absconded, via the juvenile court which had placed him on a 28-day order for emergency psychological assessment with a provision for accommodation in order to restrict his liberty. The patient had a history of absconding from placements, a criminal history involving property offences and was assessed to be a risk both to himself and to others.

It was recorded that the patient had three siblings and that his father had left home when he was a baby. One of his siblings had been brought up in a children's home and one had a history of overdosing. This patient's mother had reportedly been unable to cope with his aggressive behaviour and as a result he had been taken into care in 1989.

The patient had attended an ordinary school until he was 10. He had then been expelled for fighting with other pupils and with the teachers. He attended a number of other schools but was persistently involved in glue-sniffing, drinking and truanting. He was placed with foster parents, but was very aggressive and subsequently a care order was made. He was moved first to a children's home and then to a special needs boarding school.

During this time the patient was persistently in trouble and was eventually accused of the rape of a young girl at the school. He then absconded and went to his grandmother's home where he assaulted her so severely that she had to be admitted to hospital.

Patient 27 was admitted to Stockton Hall from court for psychological assessment. He remained there for 11 days at which time a place became available at a crisis intervention centre in Shropshire.

Case Study 14: Patient 43

This patient was a 35-year-old female admitted from Stockton Hall's sister hospital, Kneesworth House, under s.3 MHA 1983. She was described as being a 'well known problem patient' and it was recorded that staff at Kneesworth House were greatly relieved that she had been transferred because she had posed such great management problems for them.

Patient 43 had been diagnosed as suffering from severe mental handicap due to the condition known as phenylketonuria. This is a genetic condition resulting in deficiency of an enzyme normally present in the liver and results in raised blood levels of phenylaline, a toxic substance which causes damage to the developing brain. Today this is diagnosed by the Guthrie Test, but patient 43 was born eight years before the test was introduced and suffered brain damage as a result of the condition.

She had spent most of her life in care, having first been admitted to hospital at the age of six. She was described as being 'totally unmanageable, chronically tense and hyperactive'. Later on it was recorded that she became addicted to cigarette ends and tea, would frequently tear her own clothes, bite her own arms and urinate in public.

In spite of these seemingly insurmountable problems, the patient was recorded as having made some progress over the years and that she had responded to treatment well enough that in 1981 she was transferred to a self-contained flat and was supported by a special development team from the University of Kent. This support was gradually withdrawn over a period of time until 1989 when the patient was living independently and attending her local hospital as a psychiatric outpatient. Her behaviour problems persisted however, including kicking, biting, screaming and stripping. In spite of increased medication, she did not improve and was sectioned under s.3 MHA 1983 and admitted to Kneesworth House hospital.

It was recorded that the staff at Kneesworth House found her behaviour 'extraordinarily challenging', so much so that they approached Stockton Hall regarding the possible transfer of this patient. Whilst Stockton Hall did not feel that it was an appropriate setting for her in the long term, in the short term it was willing to admit her temporarily to assess her mental and physical needs, whilst some solution to her problems was found. It was agreed that after her condition had been stabilised, she should be returned to supported housing.

Patient 43 spent 79 days at Stockton Hall and was discharged to a hostel in the community.

Case Study 15: Patient 63

Patient 63 was an 18-year-old female admitted from a social services children's home under a secure accommodation order in 1990. The patient's mother had been 16 years old when the patient was born and her marriage to the patient's father was shortlived. Her mother subsequently remarried and had three more children. Patient 63 never accepted her stepfather and her name was put on the child abuse register in 1986, following an assault by him.

In 1987 the patient reported to the social services that she was being sexually abused by her stepfather and was subsequently placed in voluntary care at a local children's home. The stepfather was given a 15 month prison sentence for indecent assault.

This patient was described as 'quite bright' but had suffered not only the problems outlined above, but also from disruptive schooling since having been in care. Steps were taken to find a foster family but this process was very slow and she became extremely agitated, moody and increasingly difficult to contain in the home. She then began to abscond.

The patient was referred to a consultant in child and adolescent psychiatry and also introduced to foster parents at the weekends, but behaved in a very difficult way when she was there. During the week, staff at the children's home struggled to contain her as her behaviour deteriorated and she began to self-abuse. This involved the patient drinking cleaning fluids, taking aspirins, swallowing small objects such as buttons and slashing her own wrists. It was decided that she needed a more structured environment but that a local psychiatric ward would not be suitable because she required constant supervision. As a result, Stockton Hall agreed to admit her whilst attempts were made to find a bed at Langton House, a facility for disturbed adolescents. The patient remained at Stockton Hall for 27 days and was then transferred to Langton House.

Case Study 16: Patient 72

Patient 72 was a 16-year-old male admitted to Stockton Hall from his local Special School in 1990 under a secure care order suffering from a condition known as De Sotos Syndrome. The patient had fallen off a wall at the age of 13 after which it was recorded that his temper loss became much worse. He was described as being of limited intellectual capacity.

The patient was an only child whose father had committed suicide when he was two years old. His mother had subsequently remarried but the patient's relationship with his stepfather was described as nonexistent. The patient had several psychiatric placements and was described as presenting a 'serious management problem'. A psychiatric report indicated that there had been a failure of the normal learning processes including socialisation and as a result, the patient had developed very poorly. He had little regard for other people, displayed manipulative and disruptive behaviour and had a tendency towards gratuitous violence on a trivial stimulus. He frequently assaulted others, often using weapons such as screwdrivers. It was thought possible that the patient was suffering from temporal lobe damage – indicative of the type of head injury he had suffered – which accounted for much of his behaviour including his outbursts of irrational rage.

The patient was diagnosed as having an untreatable behaviour disorder and possible temporal lobe epilepsy. He presented such a severe management problem, having been placed in a children's home, that he was transferred to an adolescent psychiatric assessment unit. Here, the problems of his behaviour persisted to such an extent that he was transferred to Stockton Hall. The patient spent 493 days at Stockton Hall before being transferred to a mental health hostel in Wales.

Case Study 17: Patient 89

Patient 89 was a 24-year-old male admitted to Stockton Hall under s.3 MHA 1983, from Kneesworth House hospital in 1990.

This patient had been a particularly difficult breech birth and initially suffered a seizure at 13 months after contracting the measles. After a second fit at the age of two, he was unconscious for several hours. He had been slower to learn than most children and was described at the age of six as being 'generally very fearful'.

The patient had initially been brought up in Paris where he had been examined by a professor of neurology and given some medication. His behaviour did not improve, however, and at the age of 12 he was expelled from school. His family then moved to live in the UK.

From the age of 14 until he was 18, the patient attended a special needs boarding school but frequently absconded. He was then admitted to St Andrews hospital, Northampton, for a period of 16 months but was transferred to Kneesworth House hospital as a result of his unmanageable and assaultive behaviour. The staff at Kneesworth House hospital felt they had made very little progress so the patient was transferred to Stockton Hall where he was diagnosed as having mild mental handicap and a behaviour disorder.

Patient 89 was still resident at Stockton Hall in February 1995. It was recorded that the patient had improved substantially and that his parents were 'amazed at his progress' since his transfer to Stockton Hall.

Case Study 18: Patient 93

Patient 93 was a 34-year-old female admitted to Stockton Hall in 1990 under s.3 Mental Health Act 1983, from Kneesworth House Hospital. Progress had been made with this patient, but it was felt this had reached a plateau and that she would benefit from a new environment.

The patient had very elderly and disabled parents. She also had three siblings. She had first been admitted to hospital at the age of five as a result of her destructiveness and uncontrollable rages. She had remained in hospital for the majority of her life and had been admitted not only to Kneesworth but also to St Andrews, Northampton and then to Stockton Hall. During this time she had attacked several people, including her mother.

Patient 93 was described as having poor motor control, generalised ataxia, and excessive salivation problems. She was extremely violent to staff and other patients and whilst she had been at St Andrews, several hundred incidents of violence had been recorded and she had been secluded frequently. This violence began to take the form of premeditated and cunning attacks on various individuals, including biting, scratching, punching, hair-pulling and kicking. She was also prone to self-injury.

As a result of these problems, patient 93 was transferred to Stockton Hall as a severe management problem and was still resident there in February 1995.

Case Study 19: Patient 101

Patient 101 was a 27-year-old male admitted to Stockton Hall under s.3 Mental Health Act 1983 in 1990 from a hostel in the community where he had made numerous attacks on staff and other residents.

The patient had appeared to be normal as an infant but had suffered a grand mal seizure at the age of 17 months at which point he had become entirely mute. At the age of three he was admitted to Great Ormond Street Hospital because he was having seizures every three or four weeks. His behaviour was described as very difficult and he was thought to be autistic.

During his childhood, the patient attended a Rudolph Steiner School where his difficult behaviour and emotional outbursts continued. Having spent some time at the Norvic Clinic, Norwich, patient 101 went to live in a private hostel but he was physically violent to other residents and was realistically in need of an environment which provided 24-hour care. As a result the patient was transferred to Stockton Hall and was resident there in February 1995.

Case Study 20: Patient 121

The final patient in this cohort was an 18-year-old male admitted under s.37 Mental Health Act 1983 from St Andrews Hospital in 1993. He had a history of exposing himself, touching female staff and inappropriate sexual behaviour.

The patient's mother had been married three times and had a son by each of her marriages. Patient 121 was the middle of these.

At the age of three, patient 121 had suffered a skull injury and had been in a coma for three weeks. He recovered and began attending a normal school but was expelled twice for indecent behaviour. He then attended a residential school but absconded. The school refused to have him back as a result of his indecent behaviour.

After committing a sexual assault on his aunt, patient 121 was remanded to the Social Services in 1989 and was placed in a Special School. They were unable to contain him so he was transferred to Langton House, a private psychiatric hospital for disturbed adolescents. He then sexually assaulted another patient and was transferred to St Andrew's Hospital.

Patient 121 remained at St Andrews for a year but it could not modify his behaviour and he had to be put on a 'holding ward' until another suitable placement could be found because he tried to sexually assault the female staff.

He was transferred to Stockton Hall where progress was made but as a result of following a female member of staff home, had to be transferred to Kneesworth House hospital.

Discussion

Current literature regarding the study of patients admitted to forensic institutions is limited. Literature which focuses specifically on case study profiles of a cohort of patients such as this is nonexistent. This type of detailed examination is useful not only in providing an insight into this population, its characteristics and source, but also in terms of its impact on the premise that private medium secure psychiatric provision is meeting a national need not fully met by the existing public sector psychiatric provision.

The patients described in this study were initially identified as being 'of exceptional difficulty' in terms of management because they posed problems such as repetitive, assaultive or self-injurious behaviour. It was proposed that difficulties of this nature, together with resource implications and a lack of available beds in the parent district, were some of the reasons which had provided the impetus for patients' Local Health Authorities to fund a private bed. At the stage when this suggestion was made, however, this was in the main only an impression.

What this study appears to demonstrate, having focused on this sample of patients, is that this impression appears to have been borne out by further study. The 20 patients all appear to have 'long term, difficult to manage' status or are described as 'presenting severe problems of management' for their parent facilities. Although no specific reference has been made (for reasons of confidentiality) to the exact locations from where these patients came, their sources were many and varied and this suggests that Stockton Hall is meeting a national need in terms of the provision of this type of care for patients whose problems of management are documented as being outside the resource capabilities of their own regional health service facilities.

These patients also display some interesting general characteristics. These include a history of mental illness in the family, premature birth or birth defects leading to retarded development. They also display a generalised pattern of unstable home lives, periods in care or a general history of institutionalised life, often without the support of their families. A significant number have broken homes, a fact which ties in with recent research suggesting a 50 per cent rise in the prevalence of mental illness amongst children, caused by family breakdown and poor parenting (*The Times*, 19 March 1995). There also appears to be some mental illness caused by substance abuse. Most of these patients displayed violent and threatening behaviour to others which increased the problems of management which they posed in their parent district.

The response recorded in these profiles suggests an increased flexibility in the admission of such patients where no suitable regional provision was available, either because of a lack of beds, because of rejection from local facilities or because of a lack of resources needed to cater for long-term patients posing exceptional management difficulties. A cautionary note must be made, however, in the sense that the funding provided by patients' Local Health Authorities could also be seen as a significant incentive for the private sector. However, it is also documented that in many cases, Stockton Hall was successful in making progress in the treatment of these patients and in being able to discharge to suitable, often less secure, environments. It is also documented that there was a willingness to operate as a 'stop-gap' in the resettlement of patients, where another, more suitable placement was thought necessary.

This study demonstrates that in terms of access, there may be an increased flexibility in the types of patient which the private sector is prepared to admit, not only in terms of NHS referrals, but also in terms of a variety of referrals from the community and elsewhere. Obviously this is something which could be said to be driven by the demands of market forces, an issue to which the private sector is more sensitive. However, it also displays to some extent, inadequacies of the public sector in the provision of medium secure beds, of which there is a documented shortfall.

The following chapter will review these findings, together with those in chapters 5 and 6 and will outline the disparities in patient access to the public and private sectors and the motivating forces which may explain these variations.

8   Public, Private or Pluralism?
The Contributions of the
Public and Private Sectors to
Medium Secure Psychiatric
Care in the 1990s

The aim of this chapter is to review the findings of the studies described in
chapters 5, 6 and 7. It considers the differences in patient access to public and
private sector psychiatric care and discusses the motivating factors which
account for these variations. It reviews the respective contributions of the
public and private sectors in the sphere of mental health and addresses the
issue of whether a pluralistic approach to the provision of mental health care
currently exists.

Earlier chapters have outlined the development of both the Regional Secure
Unit and the more recent private psychiatric hospital. In the case of the Regional
Secure Unit, the concept had been initiated by the need for local, medium
secure psychiatric care in order to take the pressure for beds away from the
overcrowded Special Hospitals and National Health Service wards, and to
remove the mentally ill from prisons. In spite of this there has always been a
documented shortfall in the numbers of medium secure psychiatric beds
available. This has left a gap in the market that companies with experience of
providing private psychiatric care abroad have been able to fill. The advent of
private psychiatric care has provoked mixed reactions and these were also
outlined earlier in this book.

Essentially however, the time for debate about whether private psychiatric
provision *should* be here is over. It *is* here. Now, the crucial questions are
those determining what contribution it is making to the national picture of
medium secure psychiatric care. Both literature and the studies described in
previous chapters highlighted areas of concern in connection with the private
provision of psychiatric care, namely those of access, profit, quality of care

and community needs. This study has sought to concentrate on the issue of access to psychiatric care in the public and private sectors and the results of the studies at Stockton Hall, the Hutton Unit and the Norvic Clinic are now reviewed. The combined tables are reproduced in this chapter in order to be close to the text, for the reader's convenience.

Review of the Findings

Demographic Characteristics

The findings of all three studies in the area of demographic characteristics are fairly unremarkable. Stockton Hall had a slightly higher female population and more patients under the age of 20 than the Hutton Unit or the Norvic Clinic.

Table 8.1 Demographic characteristics

Age	Hutton Unit		Norvic Clinic		Stockton Hall	
Under 20			6	(7%)	13	(9%)
20–29	33	(40%)	37	(40%)	75	(53%)
3–39	28	(33%)	30	(32%)	39	(38%)
40–49	19	(22%)	19	(20%)	12	(8%)
50 and over	4	(5%)	1	(1%)	3	(2%)

Ethnic origin	Hutton Unit		Norvic Clinic		Stockton Hall	
UK	7	(94%)	85	(91%)	119	(84%)
Caribbean			1	(1%)	10	(7%)
Other European	1	(1%)	1	(1%)	1	(1%)
African	2	(2%)	6	(7%)	7	(5%)
Asian	2	(2%)			5	(3%)
No data	1	(1%)				

Gender	Hutton Unit		Norvic Clinic		Stockton Hall	
Male	76	(91%)	79	(85%)	113	(80%)
Female	8	(9%)	14	(15%)	29	(20%)

Source of Admission

Table 8.2 illustrates that in terms of referrals from either secure or non-secure facilities, Stockton Hall had a similar profile to that of the Norvic Clinic. Stockton Hall admitted 51 per cent of patients from secure facilities and 49 per cent from non-secure facilities. The Norvic Clinic admitted 43 per cent of its patients from secure facilities and 55 per cent from non-secure facilities. The Hutton Unit had a higher percentage of referrals from secure facilities (73 per cent) and only 22 per cent from non-secure facilities. This could be explained by the fact that the Hutton Unit took a significantly larger number of referrals from prison than either Stockton Hall or the Norvic Clinic. This was 48 (57 per cent) patients referred from prison to the Hutton unit compared with 31 (34 per cent) at the Norvic Clinic and 32 (23 per cent) patients at Stockton Hall.

Table 8.2 also illustrates that Stockton Hall took a larger proportion of referrals from National Health Service wards, other Regional Secure Units and police cells than either the Hutton Unit or the Norvic Clinic. This data appears to support the view that the Regional Secure Units are fulfilling the role for which they were intended in relieving pressure on prisons, NHS wards and the community, whilst also suggesting that Stockton Hall was admitting patients from a similarly wide range of sources.

Other observations were made regarding the circumstances under which patients were referred to Stockton Hall. Fifty-nine patients had been classified as either 'unmanageable' or an 'exceptional management problem' in their parent district before referral to Stockton Hall. Of these, at least 17 had been

Table 8.2   Source of Admission

		Hutton Unit		Norvic Clinic		Stockton Hall	
Secure facilities	Prison	48	(57%)	31	(34%)	32	(23%)
	RSU	1	(1%)	2	(2%)	13	(9%)
	Private hospital					7	(5%)
	Special hospital	11	(13%)	3	(3%)	5	(3%)
	Police cells	2	(2%)	5	(5%)	12	(9%)
	Secure juvenile					3	(2%)
Total		62	(73%)	41	(44%)	72	(51%)
Non-secure facilities	NHS	12	(15%)	6	(7%)	50	(36%)
	Community	10	(12%)	46	(49%)	18	(12%)
	Children's home					2	(1%)
Total		22	(27%)	52	(56%)	70	(49%)

rejected by other Regional Secure Units or Special Hospitals before being accepted by Stockton Hall. This led to further study of this cohort of patients which was described in chapter 7. This was the most significant difference between Stockton Hall, the Hutton unit and the Norvic Clinic and merits further discussion later in this chapter.

Authority for Detention

Table 8.3 demonstrates broadly similar results. The Hutton Unit and the Norvic Clinic had no patients detained under the Criminal Procedure (Insanity) Act 1964. Stockton Hall had no patients detained under sections 2, 47 or 48 of the Mental Health Act 1983. Formal patients numbered 79 (94 per cent) at the Hutton Unit, 70 (75 per cent) at the Norvic Clinic and 120 (84 per cent) at Stockton Hall. The total informal patients numbered two (two per cent) at the Hutton Unit, 19 (21 per cent) at the Norvic Clinic and 22 (16 per cent) at Stockton Hall.

Table 8.3   Authority for detention

			Hutton Unit		Norvic Clinic		Stockton Hall	
Formal patients	Part 2 MHA 1983	Section 2	4	(5%)	3	(3%)		
		Section 3	11	(13%)	7	(8%)	56	(39%)
	Part 3 MHA 1983	Section 35	10	(12%)	31	(33%)	3	(2%)
		Section 37	6	(7%)	16	(17%)	32	(22%)
		Section 37/41	12	(14%)	2	(2%)	15	(11%)
		Section 38	2	(2%)	1	(1%)	1	(1%)
		Section 47	7	(8%)	1	(1%)		
		Section 47/49	7	(8%)	5	(6%)	4	(3%)
		Section 48	12	(14%)	1	(1%)		
		Section 48/49	8	(10%)	3	(3%)	6	(4%)
		C.P.I.					3	(2%)
Total formal patients			79	(94%)	70	(75%)	120	(84%)
Informal patients			2	(2%)	19	(21%)	22	(16%)
No data			3	(4%)	4	(4%)		
Total informal patients			2	(2%)	19	(21%)	22	(16%)

Psychiatric Diagnosis

Table 8.4 demonstrates that Stockton Hall admitted more patients with a psychiatric diagnosis of either schizophrenia or psychopathy than the Hutton Unit or the Norvic Clinic. Forty-eight (34 per cent) Stockton Hall patients were diagnosed as schizophrenic compared with 33 (40 per cent) Hutton Unit patients and 28 (30 per cent) Norvic Clinic patients. Nineteen (14 per cent) Stockton Hall patients were diagnosed as psychopaths compared with three (three per cent) Norvic Clinic patients. No patients at the Hutton Unit had this diagnosis.

One other difference was that Stockton Hall had no patients detained who were diagnosed as having either a personality or mood disorder or depression, whereas the Hutton Unit had 17 (20 per cent) patients diagnosed with a personality disorder and 16 (19 per cent) with mood disorder/depression and the Norvic Clinic had 20 (22 per cent) patients with personality disorder and three (three per cent) with mood disorder/depression.

Table 8.4   Psychiatric diagnosis

	Hutton Unit		Norvic Clinic		Stockton Hall	
Schizophrenia	9	(11%)	28	(30%)	38	(27%)
Paranoid schizophrenia	24	(29%)			10	(7%)
Paranoid state	1	(1%)	5	(6%)	2	(1%)
Personality disorder	17	(20%)	20	(22%)		
Psychosis	18	(19%)			9	(6%)
Drug psychosis	6	(7%)	2	(2%)		
Depression	16	(19%)	3	(3%)		
Psychopathy			3	(3%)	19	(14%)
Organic state	1	(1%)	2	(2%)	3	(2%)
Neurosis	1	(1%)	2	(2%)		
Mental impairment	7	(9%)	2	(2%)	35	(25%)
Schizo-affective disorder	1	(1%)				
Chronic alcoholism			1	(1%)		
No diagnosis			6	(7%)		
No data	1	(1%)	1	(1%)	26	(18%)

Criminal History

In terms of criminal history the profiles are broadly similar. Patients with no previous convictions numbered 46 (33 per cent) at Stockton Hall, 19 (23 per cent) at the Hutton Unit and 30 (32 per cent) at the Norvic Clinic. The Hutton Unit and Norvic Clinic detained more patients with multiple convictions than Stockton Hall. These were 11 (13 per cent) patients at the Hutton Unit, 26 (28 per cent) at the Norvic Clinic and two (one per cent) at Stockton Hall. Stockton Hall had slightly more patients with convictions for either attempted murder or murder. This was four (three per cent) patients convicted of attempted murder and three (two per cent) patients convicted of murder. The Hutton Unit admitted one patient convicted of attempted murder and one patient convicted of murder, whereas the Norvic Clinic admitted one patient convicted of murder and no patients convicted of attempted murder.

Table 8.5   Criminal history

	Hutton Unit		Norvic Clinic		Stockton Hall	
None	19	(23%)	30	(32%)	46	(33%)
Property	18	(21%)	14	(15%)	22	(15%)
Criminal damage	8	(10%)	6	(7%)	20	(14%)
Manslaughter	1	(1%)				
Attempted murder	1	(1%)	4	(3%)		
Murder	1	(1%)	1	(1%)	3	(2%)
Sexual offences	4	(5%)	5	(5%)	14	(10%)
Nonsexual violence	9	(11%)	7	(8%)	26	(18%)
Property and sexual offences	1	(1%)				
Property and nonsexual offences	4	(5%)				
Multiple	11	(13%)	26	(28%)	2	(1%)
No data	7	(8%)	4	(4%)	5	(4%)

Previous Institutional/Psychiatric Care

Table 8.6 illustrates that the Hutton Unit and the Norvic Clinic admitted patients who had previously had contact with a much wider range of institutions than those admitted to Stockton Hall. Twenty-eight (33 per cent) Hutton Unit patients and 20 (22 per cent) Norvic Clinic patients were previously admitted to two or more other facilities. A broadly similar number of patients had been admitted to a Special Hospital previous to admission to any of the psychiatric hospitals in this study. Stockton Hall had a slightly higher number of patients who had previously been in prison or in a National Health Service psychiatric ward. This was 42 (30 per cent) Stockton Hall patients, 10 (12 per cent) Hutton Unit patients and 23 (24 per cent) Norvic Clinic patients who had previously been in prison and 43 (30 per cent) Stockton Hall patients, 22 (26 per cent) Hutton Unit patients and 17 (18 per cent) Norvic Clinic patients who had previously been in a National Health service psychiatric ward.

Table 8.6   Previous institutional/psychiatric care

	Hutton Unit		Norvic Clinic		Stockton Hall	
None	10	(12%)	10	(11%)	6	(4%)
Prison	10	(12%)	23	(24%)	42	(30%)
Special hospital	9	(11%)	5	(6%)	10	(7%)
RSU	3	(4%)	13	(14%)	6	(4%)
NHS	22	(26%)	17	(18%)	43	(30%)
Special school	2	(2%)	2	(2%)	21	(15%)
Private hospital			3	(3%)	13	(9%)
Prison and RSU	2	(2%)	6	(7%)		
Prison and special school	2	(2%)	2	(4%)		
Prison and NHS	7	(9%)	5	(6%)		
Prison, RSU and special hospital			1	(1%)		
RSU and special school			2	(2%)		
NHS and special school	4	(5%)				
RSU and special hospital	3	(4%)				
NHS and special hospital	2	(2%)				
Special hospital and special school	1	(1%)				
RSU and NHS			1	(1%)		
Prison, RSU and special school			1	(1%)		
Prison, RSU and special hospital	1	(1%)				
NHS, RSU and special hospital	1	(1%)				
RSU, special hospital and special school	1	(1%)				
Youth detention			1	(1%)		
Adolescent unit			1	(1%)		
No data	4	(5%)			1	(1%)

Discharge Details

In terms of the level of security to which patients were discharged, Stockton Hall discharged a greater number of patients to less secure environments than either the Hutton Unit or the Norvic Clinic. For Stockton Hall, the discharge of 53 patients to less secure facilities was equivalent to 72 per cent of the total discharges made at the time of the study. In comparison the Hutton Unit discharged 46 (55 per cent) patients and the Norvic Clinic 41 (44 per cent) patients to less secure facilities/environments. Similarly, the Hutton Unit and the Norvic Clinic discharged more patients to more secure facilities than Stockton Hall. This was 21 (25 per cent) patients at the Hutton Unit and 45 (48 per cent) patients at the Norvic Clinic, compared with three (four per cent of the total discharges) patients at Stockton Hall.

Table 8.7   Discharge details

		Hutton Unit		Norvic Clinic		Stockton Hall	
Less secure facilities	NHS	26	(31%)	24	(26%)	32	(22%)
	Community	20	(24%)	17	(18%)	21	(15%)
		46	(55%)	41	(44%)	53	(37%)
Same level security	RSU	2	(2%)	2	(2%)	14	(10%)
	Private hospital			4	(4%)	4	(3%)
	Special unit	1	(1%)				
		3	(3%)	6	(7%)	18	(13%)
More secure facilities	Prison	9	(11%)	40	(42%)	1	(1%)
	Special hospital	12	(14%)	5	(6%)	2	(1%)
		21	(25%)	45	(48%)	3	(2%)
	Current patients	4	(4%)			68	(48%)

Again it would be difficult to determine whether any of these results are significant without further analysis. Therefore the combined composite variables of the Hutton Unit and the Norvic Clinic were compared with those of Stockton Hall in the cases where this was statistically possible. The critic may say why combine the data from the Hutton Unit and the Norvic Clinic when they are different from each other? However, the reason for this was that it was the only simple way in which to compare RSU with the private sector.

Using observed and expected frequencies the results were again tested using the chi-square distribution. As previously mentioned, this measures the discrepancy between the frequencies and if the value of chi-square is greater than the critical value of chi-square, the result is taken to be significant. The results of this testing is as follows.

Observed and Expected Frequencies

Demographic Characteristics

Table 8.8 demonstrates that Stockton Hall takes significantly more patients under 30 years of age than either the Hutton Unit or the Norvic Clinic. Here, the chi-square is 16.79 and the critical is 14.9 (4df), so $p<0.005$. This means that the result is reliable and that there is a significant difference in the ages of patients admitted to Stockton Hall as compared to the RSUs.

Table 8.8   Demographic characteristics

Age	Hutton Unit and Norvic Clinic		Stockton Hall	
Under 20	6	(10.6)	13	(8.4)
20–29	70	(80.4)	75	(63.6)
30–39	58	(53.6)	39	(42.4)
40–49	38	(27.9)	12	(22.1)
50–59	5	(4.5)	3	(3.5)

Ethnic origin	Hutton Unit and Norvic Clinic		Stockton Hall	
UK	163	(155.9)	119	(124.1)
Other	13	(20.1)	23	(15.9)

In terms of the ethnic origin of patients, the results demonstrate that Stockton Hall admits less United Kingdom (Caucasian) patients and more patients of other ethnic origin than an RSU. The chi-square here is 6.41 and the critical level is 5.02 (1df), so p< 0.025. The result is reliable.

Authority for Detention

Table 8.9 illustrates that in terms of detention under the Mental Health Act 1983, more patients were admitted to Stockton Hall under s.3 (admission to hospital for treatment) and s.37 (the hospital order) than the RSUs and significantly less than the RSUs under s.35 (remand to hospital for reports) and s.48 (admission to hospital of other prisoners). The chi-square for this is 82.27 (9df) and p<0.001. This result appears to demonstrate that Stockton Hall admits more patients on the basis of their assessment or treatment needs than the RSUs.

Criminal History

Table 8.10 demonstrates the recorded criminal histories of the patients involved in the study. Looking at the comparison here, the chi-square is 35.84 (7df) and p<0.001. By inspection this shows that the Hutton Unit and the Norvic Clinic have significantly more patients with a criminal history including multiple conviction than those patients admitted to Stockton Hall. It does appear somewhat unusual that Stockton Hall has so few patients with multiple

Table 8.9   Authority for detention

	Hutton Unit and Norvic Clinic		Stockton Hall	
Section 3	18	(41.1)	56	(32.9)
Section 37	22	(30)	32	(24)
Section 37/41	14	(16.1)	15	(12.9)
Section 47	8	(4.4)	0	(3.6)
Section 47/49	12	(8.9)	4	(7.1)
Section 35	41	(23.9)	2	(19.1)
Section 38	2	(1.7)	1	(1.3)
Section 48	13	(7.2)	0	(5.8)
Section 48/49	11	(9.4)	6	(7.6)

Table 8.10   Criminal history

	Hutton Unit and Norvic Clinic		Stockton Hall	
Property	37	(32.7)	22	(26.3)
Criminal damage	14	(18.9)	20	(15.1)
Manslaughter	1	(0.6)	0	(0.4)
Attempted murder	1	(2.8)	4	(2.2)
Murder	2	(2.8)	3	(2.2)
Sexual offence	10	(13.3)	14	(10.7)
Nonsexual	20	(25.5)	26	(20.5)
Multiple	37	(21.6)	2	(17.4)

convictions and by inspection, far fewer than might have been expected (two as compared with the 17.4 expected). It is difficult to explain this but my impression, having collected the data, was that the medical records kept at Stockton Hall were not as complete as they might have been and this may provide some explanation for this rather large discrepancy.

Discharge Details

Table 8.11 illustrates the level of security at discharge of the patients from the Hutton Unit and the Norvic Clinic (combined) as compared with Stockton Hall. Here, the chi-square is 41.61 (2df) and p<0.001. This demonstrates quite significantly that Stockton Hall discharges far fewer patients to higher security facilities than do the RSUs.

Table 8.11   Discharge details

Level of security	Hutton Unit and Norvic Clinic		Stockton Hall	
Lower	87	(96.1)	53	(43.9)
Same	9	(18.5)	18	(8.5)
Higher	66	(47.3)	3	(21.6)

Discussion

It was outlined in chapter 3 that ownership-related trends may have important implications for mental health policy in terms of its impact upon the service being provided. The main concerns related to access, profit, quality of care and community needs.

This study has sought to concentrate on one of these concerns – that of access – although this cannot entirely be divorced from the other issues which necessarily also have an impact upon access to some extent and which will also be discussed. It was suggested at the outset that the financial pressures on private psychiatric hospitals might force a process of selectivity stemming from the need to keep empty beds to a minimum and also from the requirement of funding expensive beds in the private sector.

American literature has highlighted the possibility of manipulation of access to private hospitals. Dorwat and Schlesinger (1984) suggested that screening of patients on the basis of their ability to pay might be a problem. Similarly, Bruns and Stoudemire (1990) illustrate tight controls on access and the use of admission criteria in one profit-making psychiatric hospital as a means of achieving a 'profitable' mix of patients.

This study has sought to determine whether similar pressures to those described in the American literature also force a process of selectivity in terms of psychiatric provision in the United Kingdom. Having reviewed the general findings of the studies, the results show that although some of the findings appear unremarkable and are broadly similar, in respect of the source of patients and the details recorded concerning their admission to these hospitals, there is some variation which merits further discussion. These differences can be explained by suggesting that a process of selectivity operates in relation to patient access to both the public and private sectors, but with differing motivating forces. This examination focuses on that selectivity and how other issues such as profit and community needs also impact upon this.

In respect of the findings at the Hutton Unit and the Norvic Clinic, chapter 5 suggested that the characteristics of patients admitted to the Hutton Unit and the Norvic Clinic were broadly similar in nature, as were the sources of referral and the circumstances (when recorded) in which admissions were made. They accepted referrals from quite a wide range of sources, both secure and non-secure and appeared to be fulfilling the role for which they were intended. This was outlined earlier in the same chapter as being a pressure-relieving facility for the overcrowded Special Hospitals, National Health Service psychiatric wards and prisons. In terms of these referrals, they could also be seen to be providing a service to the community in which they were situated.

In respect of the Stockton Hall admission study, it was outlined in chapter 6 that the growth of private medium secure psychiatric care was a response to a national shortage of medium secure beds within the public sector. This was thought to relate in particular to patients who may require this type of care on a protracted basis and initially this suggestion was merely an impression.

Although the study showed some similarities with the Hutton Unit and the Norvic Clinic in that Stockton Hall accepted referrals from quite a wide range of sources, it also demonstrated some interesting features of the admission population which were not evident from the data collected at either the Hutton Unit or the Norvic Clinic. This was that a significant number of patients admitted to Stockton Hall had been identified, in their parent district, as being of exceptional difficulty in terms of the management problems which they posed. It was these difficulties, often long-term in nature, which appeared to motivate their referral to Stockton Hall. In the 59 cases identified, Stockton Hall was apparently prepared to admit patients referred by their parent facilities because of long-term management problems or those who had been rejected by their parent facilities, usually for the same reason. This disparity in patient access to the public and private sectors is an interesting feature which merits further investigation.

In relation to access to the public sector, this reflects the absence of long-term medium secure provision, with Regional Secure Units only being prepared to accept patients who require their services for two years or less. Therefore, patients who pose exceptional management problems are most likely to be long-term patients and not those whom Regional Secure Units are willing to admit.

This illustrates a lack of resources in the National Health Service resulting in Regional Secure Units not only having a limited number of beds available, but also selectively screening out patients whose problems of management are likely to be long-term and who pose a drain on their resources. The result is that for patients of this sort, their needs are not being met within their parent district and subsequently, the existence of private medium secure care makes it possible for RSUs to reject unmanageable patients in order for the more well-resourced private sector to pick them up. This of course depends on the necessary funding being provided by the Local Health Authority or, more recently, the purchasing authority in question. This process of selectivity is therefore motivated by a lack of resources as well as a documented shortfall in available medium secure beds. Other factors may also have a bearing on this.

It was noted in previous chapters that the idea of the Regional Secure Unit was first recommended by the Butler Committee (1975). The Committee also recommended that Regional Secure Units should not necessarily provide long-term psychiatric hospitalisation for the chronically mentally ill, but the sort of care a patient might need for a period of two years or less. When the Committee made this recommendation it was simply that, it was not mandatory, but a suggestion of the type of care it foresaw the units providing. I have been informed by forensic psychiatrists working within the system, that since this time, a culture has grown in the Regional Secure Units whereby they have taken on board the suggestion made by the Butler Committee (1975) by being extremely reluctant to admit those patients likely to be long-term because these patients obviously pose the most problems and are the most difficult to treat. The culture is therefore, that beds will be filled with easier patients if possible and those patients likely to be long-term are considered later. This has created a gap in the market for more long-term medium secure psychiatric provision, which is now being filled by independent providers such as Partnerships in Care. This is a lucrative gap in the market. How lucrative can be demonstrated by the fact that the most current trend within the public sector is that NHS trusts are now starting to provide private beds which they are selling on the open market, at the same price as those offered by independent providers. The profit motive in this sense has pre-empted more competition between the public and the private sectors.

Another issue which these findings illustrate is that whilst the lack of beds and resources in the public sector apparently creates an inability and, to some extent, an unwillingness to provide for certain patients, it does not (at least for some Local Health Purchasing Authorities) prevent the funding of expensive beds in the private sector. Does this indicate the success of the private sector in the quality provision of psychiatric services on which the public sector can rely or does it reflect the failure, in terms of fiscal management or clinical provision, of the public sector? There is one other alternative. Perhaps it represents the acknowledgement of both sectors of the advantages to be gained, in a less than perfect system, from working towards an essentially pluralistic system of psychiatric provision in which both have a role to play and both stand to benefit from this sort of cooperation. To understand this more fully it is necessary to describe in more detail the provision of regional psychiatric care and how such contracts are entered into by Health Authorities and psychiatric providers.

Currently, there are no standard contracts for the provision of psychiatric care at regional level. Government funding is given directly to each region's Local Health Purchasing Authority. The purchasing authority then makes its own blanket contracts with a number of hospitals, who, for a given sum, agree to provide such psychiatric care as that region's patients are likely to require. The contract is therefore between the purchasing authority and the hospital. If it is the case that subsequently, a Regional Secure Unit refuses to admit, or readmit a difficult patient, the purchasing authority must then find an alternative, and what is more, pay for that alternative. Having already paid once for its contract for psychiatric provision with the RSU, the purchasing authority then ends up paying a further sum to an independent provider, if that is where the patient ends up. This process benefits RSUs in that they relieve themselves of the most difficult patients, and can justify this by reference to the suggestions of the Butler Committee (1975). It also benefits independent providers because they can then enter a lucrative contract with the purchasing authority for admitting the patient.

This is not to say, however, that independent providers like Stockton Hall always fill their beds with the most difficult patients. They too will fill their beds with easier patients if at all possible, but logic suggests that if they have empty beds they *will* fill them with more serious patients in order not to lose money.

This appears to demonstrate that a process of selectivity is prevalent both in the public and private sectors.

In terms of the Stockton Hall studies described in chapters 6 and 7 they demonstrate an increased flexibility in the admission of 'unmanageable' patients, where it is documented that no suitable regional provision was available. The data collected from these studies not only implies a process of selectivity operated by the public sector in rejecting patients who are a drain on resources, but also demonstrates that a significant number of these types of patients are referred to and accepted by Stockton Hall. Chapter 7 illustrates a cohort of 59 patients identified in this way who were accepted and largely successfully treated by Stockton Hall, as the detailed case studies show.

It has been demonstrated that referral to a private psychiatric hospital is a good business opportunity for the accepting facility. The profit to be made from providing private beds for these patients is not insignificant and must provide an incentive for an independent provider such as Stockton Hall. Private psychiatric care is expensive and chapter 4 outlined this cost (at the time of the study) as being in excess of £200 per patient per day. Because Stockton Hall is a profit-making facility, it cannot accept patients unless the necessary funding is in place. Indeed, the medical files of a number of the patients to which I had access recorded delays in finalising the referral of some patients resulting from difficulties in clarifying the funding of a bed by the Purchasing Authority in question. This suggests that a process of selectivity is prevalent in the private sector also, but unlike the public sector, it is the demands of market forces which pre-empt this selectivity. Stockton Hall is willing and able to take difficult and potentially long-term patients, as long as the appropriate funding is in place.

Profit must therefore play a large part in the provision of private secure care but does it mean that the quality of care provided is inadequate? It was documented in many cases that Stockton Hall made progress in the treatment of many of its patients, who were subsequently discharged to suitable, often less secure, accommodation. It is also recorded that they were willing to act as a 'stop-gap' in the resettlement of patients who required other suitable accommodation which could not be found immediately. The ability to cope with these situations is, in part, a result of greater resources than are prevalent in the public sector. It suggests that realistically, fiscal considerations do affect the organisational behaviour of the public and private sectors. What remains uncertain because of a lack of research, is whether the respective contributions of the public and private sectors are affected beneficially or detrimentally by the profit motive.

In this respect, further research must be carried out to evaluate and monitor this. The problems associated with effectively measuring quality of care however, were outlined in chapter 3. It is also necessary to have the full cooperation of the psychiatric providers involved. My own experience was that although public and private providers realised the mutual benefits of the system as it currently exists, there was also an element of suspicion on the part of Stockton Hall combined with a leaning towards secrecy in relation to the regime operated there. My own research at Stockton Hall was initially made possible and encouraged by two forensic psychiatrists working there who subsequently moved back into the public sector. Having collected some information at Stockton Hall, both psychiatrists left and access to patient medical files had to be renegotiated at great length. Although I was eventually allowed to return to Stockton Hall two years later to collect further information for the case studies described in chapter 7, it was made fairly clear that because I was also researching and having contact with several other Regional Secure Units, one of which was where the two psychiatrists previously employed at Stockton Hall now worked, that no other information would be made available to me. I count myself very fortunate to have collected the data I subsequently did and in defence of my methodology, whilst more issues could have been examined, perhaps particularly that of applications, the research that was done was the best which could be achieved under the circumstances.

In respect of quality of care which is essentially a difficult concept to measure in relation to mental health care, where there is an absence of structural measures, it has been demonstrated that whilst market forces are prevalent in terms of the fact that referrals to Stockton Hall did receive prompt attention, the deciding factor in admission had to be the willingness of the patient's Local Health Purchasing Authority to fund the bed. In this situation it is the Purchasing Authority who is the customer and not the patient and the quality of care provided by Stockton Hall must be of interest to the authority in question. However, the fact that Stockton Hall accepts referrals from regional psychiatric hospitals all over the country makes it more difficult to address the issue of the quality of care being provided because of the very nature of patients being dislocated from their own, often far-flung parent districts.

This fact also raises the issue of community needs. Stockton Hall (like other private hospitals) does not primarily serve the community in which it is located, unlike Regional Secure Units which were intended to perform this role. Stockton Hall therefore fits into the psychiatric picture of care on a national, rather than a regional basis. This has an impact on the issue of community needs and clearly distinguishes the private from the public sector influence in this respect. There are problems associated with providing psychiatric care on this basis in that dislocation from the patient's home area and the referring Health Authority mean that continuation of care and follow-up after discharge must be very difficult, if they are possible at all. In this sense too it is extremely difficult to address the issue of quality of care and more research is needed to clarify these issues.

One possibility would be an intensive interview study of decision-makers who decide to place patients either in a Regional Secure Unit or at Stockton Hall. The fact that Stockton Hall patients are often said to be unmanageable may, after all have a simple explanation. People at the sending end may have to describe them in those terms to unlock the coffers, and the label sticks. For this reason a study of decision-makers would be timely.

A factor which has probably also provided at least some of the impetus for the private provision of psychiatric services in this country is the process of deinstitutionalisation which has been ongoing for about 40 years, but which has accelerated in the last decade. Just as Schlesinger and Dorwat (1984) attribute the growth in private psychiatric hospitals in America to an increased need for psychiatric beds arising from the state policy of deinstitutionalisation, the gap in the market for secure psychiatric beds in the United Kingdom can be attributed to a similar trend together with the admission culture of RSUs which has grown from the recommendations of the Butler Committee (1975) and which has already been described. The reduction in the number of psychiatric beds available in the United Kingdom in favour of what the government has called 'community care' has had many justifications. Most famous perhaps in relation to this were the ideologies of Michel Foucault who saw the development of psychiatric hospitals not as a humane approach, but as an extension of the repressive apparatus of the bourgeois state. In this sense, the psychiatric insti-tution (the asylum) was just a means of segregating difficult members of society and worked also as a warning to others. This, together with the idea of bleak wards filled with wandering patients, provides a powerful emotional message.

From ideologies such as this came the notion and thereafter the policy of 'care in the community'. Not only a good idea from the point of view of closing down asylums, but also in terms of fiscal feasibility. It has since become evident however, that the community can be a less then welcoming place where the mentally ill often suffer from isolation, squalor and homelessness and where those in the community also suffer – a fact which the likes of Jonathan Newby and John Zito found to their cost.[1] Now, finding a psychiatric bed has become a time-consuming bureaucratic nightmare for doctors and the gap in the market for private providers which this has produced gets bigger. Perhaps the advent of the private psychiatric hospital means that we have merely come full circle and that in this sense, sanity really is a return to the (private) asylum (Dalrymple, 1995).

Conclusion

In terms of the respective contributions of the public and private sectors in the field of medium secure psychiatric care, this study has shown that, broadly speaking, Regional Secure Units like the Hutton Unit and the Norvic Clinic are fulfilling the role for which they were intended. This was to provide regional psychiatric care in conditions of medium security, to take the pressure for beds away from National Health Service wards and Special Hospitals, to remove the mentally ill from prisons, and to provide this service for the community in which they were situated. They appear to be doing this, but not without problems. First, there are not enough of them and this documented shortfall has been outlined. Those that exist appear to be limited in the service they can offer and to what sort of patients due to resource implications. This means that they screen out patients who pose exceptional management problems and who as a result may need psychiatric care for a period in excess of two years. Effectively, this has meant that, together with the policy of deinstitutionalisation favoured by the government, this has produced a substantial gap in the market of which private, overseas providers have sought to take advantage. The incentive to step in and provide this type of psychiatric care is primarily financial and there continues to be a need for it in the current climate.

This study has demonstrated that Local Health Purchasing Authorities could be said to be in a 'cleft stick' over the provision of this type of psychiatric care. Regional Secure Units appear to provide as much for local patients as their resources will allow, but this apparently does not include the capability or willingness, due to the Butler recommendations, to take on long-term difficult to manage patients. The study of Stockton Hall showed the most obvious differences from the Hutton Unit and the Norvic Clinic in respect of the fact that it was prepared to admit patients classed as 'unmanageable' or those rejected by their parent facilities. This did demonstrate the increased flexibility of Stockton Hall in terms of the patients it was willing (and able) to admit, but moreover it illustrates a process of selectivity. This selectivity is prevalent in both sectors but in the public sector is motivated by their own capabilities and resources, and the taking on board of the recommendations of the Butler Committee (1975). In the private sector the motivation is, most logically, financial.

In spite of this, it is possible to say that Stockton Hall is making an important contribution to medium secure psychiatric care. Significantly, it has been demonstrated that Stockton Hall, despite having been shown to accept a high proportion of 'unmanageable' patients does discharge far more patients to less secure facilities. Further research must however be carried out to clarify this contribution. There is a need to look closely at the quality of services being provided in the public and private sectors. There is also a need to clarify the situation regarding the lack of regional beds and inability of some Regional Secure Units to cope with difficult patients, whilst it is, at the same time apparently still possible for Local Health Purchasing Authorities to fund expensive beds in the private sector. What these apparent disparities in access between the public and private sectors in my opinion have essentially brought about is a pluralistic system of referral which operates within this sphere of health care, which, although it appears to work successfully and to benefit each side respectively, has actually been arrived at more by accident than by design.

This study demonstrates that the development of medium secure psychiatric provision within Partnerships in Care, as well as other independent operators, can be seen as a private sector, market orientated response to a national shortage of medium secure beds, in particular relating to patients identified as posing exceptional management problems within their parent district, or those requiring medium secure care on a protracted basis.

I consider that it also demonstrates that the independent sector is now becoming firmly entrenched in the speciality of forensic psychiatry and the provision of medium secure psychiatric units. It illustrates that Stockton Hall provides a broadly based psychiatric service for offender (forensic) patients and other difficult to manage patients who require this type of care and treatment. The characteristics of Stockton Hall patients are often similar to the types of patients admitted to regional Secure Units. Stockton Hall does, however, demonstrate an increased flexibility in the type of patient it is prepared to admit. In my opinion, this study has demonstrated that this flexibility is driven by the demands of market forces, which the independent sector, in order to prosper, has to be sensitive to. In this sense, the inadequacies of the National Health Service, in meeting the needs for patients requiring treatment in secure conditions continues to be an area of both need and sensitivity.

Note

1 Jonathan Newby and John Zito were both killed by schizophrenics who had been discharged into the care of the community.

Bibliography

Adam, C. et al. (1992), *Adjusting Privatization: Case Studies from Developing Countries*, London: Heinemann.

American Psychiatric Association (1995), *The Diagnostic and Statistical Manual of Mental Disorders*, 4th edn: American Psychiatric Press.

Andrews, G. (1989), 'Private and Public Psychiatry: A Comparison of Two Health Care Systems', *American Journal of Psychiatry*, 146, 7, 881–6.

Audit Commission (1986), *Making a Reality of Community Care*, London: HMSO.

Allam, D.P. (1990), 'Sentencing the Mentally Disordered', *The Magistrate*, October Issue, 1990.

Adam Smith Institute (1988), *Omega Justice Project*, London: Adam Smith Institute.

Ascher, K. (1989), *The Politics of Privatisation*, London: Macmillan.

Bean, J.P. (1992), 'A Private Sort of Place', *New Law Journal*, 20, p. 1610.

Bean, J.P. (1993), 'Prisoner – Group 4', *New Law Journal*, 7 May, p. 648.

Berry, M. (1990), 'Regional Secure Units in the Emerging Picture' in Edwards, G. (ed.), *Current Issues in Clinical Psychology*, London: Plenum Press.

Blackburn, R. (1993), *The Psychology of Criminal Conduct: Theory, Research and Practice*, John Wiley & Sons: Chichester.

Borna, S. (1986), 'Free Enterprise Goes to Prison', *British Journal of Criminology*, 26, pp. 321–34.

Bos, D. (1993), 'Privatization In Europe – A Comparison of Approaches', *Oxford Review of Economic Policy*, 9, pp. 95–111.

Bowden, P. (1995), 'Confidential Inquiry into Homicides and Suicides by Mentally Ill People: A Preliminary Report on Homicide', editorial for the *Psychiatric Bulletin*, 19, pp. 65–6.

Bowden, P.R. (1983), 'The Regional Secure Unit Programme; A Personal Appraisal', *Royal College of Psychiatrists Bulletin*, 143, pp. 138–40.

Butler, E. et al. (1985), *The Omega File. A Complete Review of Government Functions*, London: Adam Smith Institute.

Butler, E. (ed.) (1990), *Privatisation Now!*, London: Adam Smith Institute.

Butler, E. et al. (1993), *But Who Will Regulate the Regulators?*, London: ASI.

Bruns, W. and Stoudemire, A. (1990), 'Development of a Medical-Psychiatric Programme within the Private Sector: Potential Problems and Strategies for their Resolution', *General Hospital Psychiatry*, 12, 3, pp. 137–47.

Camp, C. and Camp, G. (1985), 'Correctional Privatisation in Perspective', *Prison Journal*, 62, pp. 14–31.

Chan, J.B.L. (1992), 'The Privatisation of Punishment – A Review of the Key Issues', *Australian Journal of Social Issues*, 27, 4, pp. 223–47.

Cohen, S. (1985), *Visions of Social Control: Crime, Punishment and Classification*, Cambridge: Polity Press.

Cohen, S. and Scull, A. (eds) (1983), *Social Control and the State: Historical and Comparative Essays*, Oxford: Robertson.

Coid, J.W. (1988), 'Mentally Abnormal Prisoners on Remand: Rejected or Accepted by the NHS?', *British Medical Journal*, 296, pp. 1779–988.

Coid, J.W. (1991), 'A Survey of Patients from Five Health Districts Receiving Special Care in the Private Sector', *Psychiatric Bulletin*, 15, pp. 257–62.

Coid, J.W. (1993), *A Survey of Bed Occupancy in Medium Security*, unpublished paper for the Department of Health, 21 November.

Coid, J.W. (1994), 'Failure in Community Care; Psychiatry's Dilemma,' *British Medical Journal*, 308, pp. 805–6.

Cooke, A. et al. (1944), 'Something to Lose: Case Management of Mentally Disordered Offenders', *Journal of Mental Health*, 3, pp. 59–67.

Cooke, D.J. (1989), 'Containing Violent Prisoners. An Analysis of Barlinnie Special Unit', *British Journal of Criminology*, 29, p. 2.

Cowan, L.G. (1990), *Privatization in the Developing World*, New York: Praeger.

Cox, M. (1978), *Structuring the Therapeutic Process: Compromise with Chaos*, London: Jessica Kingsley Publishers (reprinted 1995).

Dalrymple, T. (1995), Sanity is a Return to the Asylums, *The Times*, 27 August.

DHSS (1974), *The Glancy Report on Security in NHS Hospitals*, London: HMSO.

DHSS (1975), *The Butler Committee Report on Mentally Abnormal Offenders*, London: HMSO, Cmnd 6244.

DiIulio, J.J. Jr. (1990), 'The Duty to Govern. A Critical Perspective on the Private Management of Prisons and Jails' in McDonald, D.C. (ed.) (1990), *Private Prisons and the Public Interest*, New Brunswick, NJ: Rutgers University Press, pp. 155–78.

DiIulio, J.J. Jr. (1990), 'Prisons for Profit', *Commentary*, pp. 66–8.

Dorwat, R., Epstein, S. and Davidson, S. (1988), 'The Shifting Balance of Public and Private Inpatient Psychiatric Services: Implications for Administrators', *Administration and Policy in Mental Health*, 16, 1, p. 4.

Dorwat, R. and Schlesinger, M. (1984), 'Ownership and Mental Health Services', *New England Journal of Medicine*, 311, 15, pp. 959–65.

Dorwat, R. and Schlesinger, M. (1988), 'Privatisation of Psychiatric Services', *American Journal of Psychiatry*, 145, 5, pp. 543–53.

Dorwat, R. et al. (1988), 'The Shifting Balance of Public and Private Inpatient Psychiatric Services: Implications for Administrators', *Administration and Policy in Mental Health*, 16, 1, pp. 4–13.

Elvin, J. (1985), 'A Civil Liberties View of Private Prisons', *Prison Journal*, 654, pp. 48–52.

Farrell, M. (ed.), (1989), *Punishment for Profit*, London: Institute for the Study and Treatment of Delinquency.

Fennel, P. (1991), 'Diversion of Mentally Disordered Offenders from Custody', *Criminal Law Review*, pp. 333–46.

Flynn, N. (1990), *Public Sector Management*, London: Harvester Wheatsheaf.

Fraser, R. and Wilson, M. (1988), *Privatization: The UK Experience and International Trends*, Keesing's International Studies, Longman Group UK.

Friedman, D. (1973), *The Machinery of Freedom: Guide to a Radical Capitalism*, New York: Harper and Row.

Friedman, M. (1962), *Capitalism and Freedom*, Chicago: Chicago University Press.

Friedman, M. (1980), *Free to Choose*, London: Secker and Warburg.

Gamble, A. (1988), *The Free Economy and the Strong State: The Politics of Thatcherism*, Macmillan Education: Basin.

Garland, D. and Young, P.V. (eds)(1989), *The Power to Punish: Contemporary Penality and Social Analysis*, Gower: Aldershot.

George, V. and Millar, S. (1990), *Social Policy Towards 2000*, London: Routledge and Kegan Paul.

Gibbens, T.C. and Robertson, G. (1983), 'A Survey of the Criminal Careers of Hospital Order Patients', *British Journal of Psychiatry*, 143, pp. 362–9.

Gibson, R.W. (1978), 'Private Psychiatric Hospitals: "Excellence is their Watchword"', *American Journal of Psychiatry*, 135, pp. 17–21.

Gostin, L. (1977), *A Human Condition: The Mental Health Act from 1959–1975*, National Association for Mental Health: London. MIND Special Report.

Gostin, L. (1985), *Secure Provision: A Review of Special Services for the Mentally Ill and Mentally Handicapped in England and Wales*, London: Tavistock.

Grounds, A. (1991), 'The Transfer of Sentenced Prisoners to Hospital 1960–1983: A Study in one Special Hospital', *British Journal of Criminology*, 31, 1.

Gudjonsson, G. and MacKeith, J.A.C. (1983), 'A Regional Interim Secure Unit at the Bethlem Royal Hospital – The First Fourteen Months', *Medicine, Science and the Law*, 23, 3, pp. 209–19.

Gunn, J. (1977), 'Criminal Behaviour and Mental Disorder', *British Journal of Psychiatry*, 130, pp. 317–29.

Gunn, J. (1978), *Psychiatric Aspects of Imprisonment*, Academic Press: London.

Hall, S. (1988), *The Hard Road to Renewal: Thatcherism and the Crisis of the Left*, London: Verso.

Hansard (1993), *The House of Commons Official Report of the Prisons (Contracting Out), Debate*, 3 May, London: HMSO, Vol. 218, No. 115.

Henry, S. (1983), *Private Justice. Towards Integrated Theorising in the Sociology of Law*, London: Routledge and Kegan Paul.

Higgins, J. (1981), 'Four Years Experience of an Interim Secure Unit', *British Medical Journal*, 282, pp. 889–93.

Hinton, J.W. (1983), *Dangerousness: Problems of Assessment and Predication*, London: Allen and Unwin.

Hobbes, T. (1991), *Leviathan*, edited by Tuck, R. *Cambridge Texts in the History of Social and Political Thought*, Cambridge: Cambridge University Press (original work published 1651).

Hoenig, F. and Hamilton, M.W. (1969), *The De-Segregation of the Mentally Ill*, London: Routledge and Kegan Paul.

Hoggett, B.M. (1984), *Mental Health Law*, 2nd edn, London: Sweet and Maxwell.

Home Office (1996), *Wolds Remand Prison – An Evaluation*, a study commissioned by the Home Office Research and Statistics Directorate, carried out by Keith Bottomley, Adrian James, Emma Clare and Alison Liebling, Research Findings No. 32, April, London: HMSO.

Home Office (1989), *Mental Health Act Commission 3rd Biennial Report 1987–1989*, chaired by Louis Blom-Cooper, 50pp, 30cm Nov. 1989, London: HMSO.

Home Office (1991), *Department of Health and Home Office Review of Health and Social Services for Mentally Disordered Offenders and Others Requiring Similar Services*, chaired by Dr J.L. Reed, London: HMSO.

Home Office (1987), *Contract Provision of Prisons*, London: HMSO.

Home Office (1988), *Private Sector Involvement in the Remand System*, HM Inspector of Prisons, Annual Report for 1986, London: HMSO, Cmnd 434.

Howard League (1987), *Prisons for Profit?*, London: Howard League.

Jeffers, J. and Britton, N. (1985), 'Some Necessary Assumptions in Psychiatric Treatment Centres: The Functions and Dysfunctions of Myths', *Psychiatric Quarterly*, 57, 1, pp. 59–71.

Johnson, C. (ed.) (1988), *Privatisation and Ownership, Vol.1*, London: Pinter.

Jones, K. (1972), *A History of the Mental Health Services*, London: Routledge and Kegan Paul.

Jones, K. and Poletti, A. (1985), 'The Italian Transformation of the Asylum: A Commentary and Review', *International Journal of Mental Health*, 14, 1–2, pp. 195–212.

Jones, R.E. (1983), 'Moral Treatment: The Basis of Private Mental Hospital Care', *Psychiatric Hospital*, 14, 1, pp. 5–9.

Kearns, A. and O'Connor, A. (1988), 'The Mentally Handicapped Criminal Offender', *British Journal of Psychiatry*, 152, pp. 848–85.

Lilly, J.R. and Knepper, P. (1992), 'An International Persective on the Privatisation of Corrections', *The Howard Journal of Criminal Justice*, 31, 3.

LeGrand, J. (1993), *Quasi-Markets and Social Policy*, London: Macmillan.

LeGrand, J. and Robinson, R. (eds) (1984), *Privatisation in the Welfare State*, London: Allen & Unwin.

Locke, J. (1955), *On Civil Government*, Chicago: Henry Regnery (original work published 1692).

Logan, C. (1990), *Private Prisons: Cons and Pros*, New York: Oxford University Press.

Mackay, R.D. and Ward, T. (1994), 'The Long-Term Detention of those found Unfit to Plead and Legally Insane', *British Journal of Criminology*, 34, 1.

Mackenzie, C. (1988), 'Psychiatry for the Rich: A History of the Private Madhouse at Ticehurst in Surrey 1792–1917', *Psychological Medicine*, 18, 3, pp. 545–9.

Maguire, M., Vagg, J. and Morgan, R. (eds) (1985), *Accountability and Prisons: Opening up a Closed World*, London: Tavistock.

Marks, I. and Thornicroft, G. (1990), 'Private Inpatient Psychiatric Care', *British Medical Journal*, 300, p. 892.

Matthews, R. (ed.) (1989), *Privatising Criminal Justice*, London:Sage.

Matthews, R. (1988), 'Making Crime Pay', *New Society*, 12 February, pp. 11–2.

McConville, S. and Hall Williams, E. (1985), *Crime and Punishment: A Radical Rethink*, London: Tawney Society.

McCue, M.J. and Clements, J.P. (1993), 'Relative Performance of For-Profit Psychiatric Hospitals in Investor Owned Systems and Non-Profit Hospitals', *American Journal of Psychiatry*, 150, 1, pp. 77–82.

McDonald, D.C. (1994), 'Public Imprisonment by Private Means: The Re-Emergence of Private Prisons and Jails in the United States, the United Kingdon and Australia', *British Journal of Criminology*, Vol. 34, Special Issue.

Ministry of Health (1961), *The Emery Report of a Working Party on the Special Hospitals Programme*, London: Ministry of Health.

Mollica, R.F. (1985), 'From Antonio Gramsci to Franco Basaglia: The Theory and Practise of the Italian Psychiatric Reform', *International Journal of Mental Health*, 14, 1–2, pp. 22–41.

Monahan, J. and Steadman, H. (1983), 'Crime and Mental Disorder: An Epidemiological Approach' in Tonry and Morris (eds), *Crime and Justice*, Vol. 4.

Morgan, R. and King, R. (1987), 'Profiting from Prison', *New Society*, 23 October.

Moyle, P. (1993), 'Privatisation of Prisons in New South Wales and Queensland: A Review of some Key Developments in Australia', *The Howard Journal of Criminal Justice*, 32, 3.

NACRO (1993), *Community Care and Mentally Disturbed Offenders*, Mental Health Advisory Committee Policy Paper No. 1, London: NACRO.

Naismith, L.J. and Coldwell, J.B. (1988), 'A Comparison of Male Admissions to a Special Hospital 1970–1971 and 1987–1988', *Medicine, Science and the Law*, 30, 4, pp. 301–8.

National Health Service (1994), 'Guidance on the Discharge of Mentally Disordered People and their Continuing Care in the Community', *Health Service Guidelines*, 94, 27.

Nozick, R. (1974), *Anarchy, State and Utopia*, New York: Basic Books.

O'Connor, J. (1984), 'Public vs. Private Responsibility for Mental Health Services', *Hospital and Community Psychiatry*, 35, 9, p. 877.

Osler, A. (1991), 'Mentally Disordered Offenders', *The Magistrate*, October.

Papadakis, E., Taylor Gooby, P. (1987), *The Private Provision of Public Welfare*, London: Harvester Wheatsheaf.

Parry, R. (1990), 'The Private Challenge for Practitioners' in Parry, R. (ed.), *Privatisation*, Research Highlights in Social Work 18, London: Jessica Kingsley Publishers Ltd.

Pease, K. and Taylor, M. (1989), 'Private Prisons and Penal Purpose' in Matthews, R. (ed.), *Privatising Criminal Justice*, London: Sage.

Prins, H. (1995), *Offenders, Deviants or Patients?*, 2nd edn, London: Routledge & Kegan Paul.

Prins, H. (1986), *Dangerous Behaviour: The Law and Mental Disorder*, London: Tavistock.

Prins, H. (1990), *Bizarre Behaviours: Boundaries of Psychiatric Disorder*, London: Tavistock.

Prins, H. (1994), 'Is Diversion Just a Diversion?', *Medicine, Science and the Law*, 34, pp. 137–47.

Prison Report (1995), 'Privatisation Factfile: Blakenhurst, Judge Tumim Reports', *Prison Report*, Spring, No. 30.

Reynolds, A. (1992), 'The Soft Cell', *New Statesman*, No. 21, 10 July.

Robertson, G. (1981), *The Extent and Pattern of Crime among Mentally Handicapped Offenders*, British Institute Mental Handbook, No. 3, pp. 100–3.

Roth, G. (1988), *The Private Provision of Public Services in Developing Countries*, London: Oxford University Press.

Royal College of Psychiatrists (1980), *Secure Facilities for Psychiatric Patients: A Comprehensive Policy*, London: Royal College of Psychiatrists.

Ryan, M. and Ward, T. (1989), *Privatization and the Penal System: The American Experience and the Debate in Britain*, Milton Keynes: Open University Press.

Sampson, A, (1991), 'Who Guards the Private Guards?', *Prison Report*, Spring.

Savage, P. and Robins, L. (eds) (1990), *Public Policy under Thatcher*, London: Macmillan.

Savas, E.S. (1982), *Privatising the Public Sector*, London: Chatham House.

Schwartz, S. et al. (1989), 'The Short-Term Treatment Unit: A Case Report of Public/Private Collaboration', *Administration and Policy in Mental Health*, 17, 2, pp. 91–100.

Sellars, M. (1993), *The History and Politics of Private Prisons*, London: Associated University Press.

Scott, P.D. (1974), Solutions to the Problem of the Dangerous Offender, *British Medical Journal*, 4, pp. 640–1.

Scull, A. (1977), *Decarceration: Community Treatment and the Deviant. A Radical View*, Englewood: Prentice-Hall.

Shichor, D. (1995), *Punishment for Profit*, London: Sage.

Sim, J. (1990), *Medical Power in Prisons: The Prison Medical Service in England 1774–1989*, Crime, Justice and Social Policy Series, Milton Keynes: Open University Press.

Smith, A. (1910), *The Wealth of Nations*, Vol. 2, London: Everyman's Library, Dent (original work published 1776).

Smith, A. (1970), *The Wealth of Nations*, Books 1–3 (reprinted), introduction by Skinner, A. Pelican Classics, Penguin: Harmondsworth (original work published 1776).

Snowden, P. (1983), 'The Regional Secure Unit Programme', *Bulletin of the Royal College of Psychiatrists*, pp. 138–41.

Snowden, P. (1985), 'A Survey of the Regional Secure Unit Programme', *British Journal of Psychiatry*, 147, pp. 499–507.

Sparks, R. (1994), 'Can Prisons be Legitimate? Penal Politics, Privatisation and the Timeliness of an Old Idea', *British Journal of Criminology*, Vol. 34, Special Issue.

Taylor, P. and Gunn, J. (1984), 'Violence and Psychosis', *British Medical Journal*, 288, pp. 1945–9.

Taylor Gooby, P. and Lawson, R. (eds) (1993), *Markets and Managers*, Open University Press.

Tennent, G. et al. (1974), 'Male Admissions to Broadmoor Hospital', *British Journal of Psychiatry*, 125, pp. 44–50.

Teplin, I. (1983), 'The Criminalisation of the Mentally Ill: Speculation and Research of Data', *Psychological Bulletin*, 94, pp. 54–67.

Tonak, D. (1992), 'Mentally Disordered Offenders and the Criminal Justice Act 1991', *Probation Journal*.

Travis, L.F. et al. (1985), 'Private Enterprise and Institutional Corrections: A Call for Caution', *Federal Probation*, 49, 4, pp. 11–6.

Treasaden, I.H. (1985), 'Current Practice in regional Interim Secure Units' in Gostin, L. (ed.), *Secure Provision: A Review of Services for the Mentally Ill and Mentally Handicapped in England and Wales*, London: Tavistock.

Veljanovski, C. (1988), *Selling the State*, London: Weidenfeld and Nicolson.

Vickers, J. and Yarrow, G. (1988), *Privatization: An Economic Analysis*, London: MIT Press.

Walker, J. and McCabe (1973), *Crime and Insanity in England and Wales*, Vol.2. Edinburgh University Press.

Walker, N. (ed.) (1996), *Dangerous People*, London: Blackstone.

Wasik, M. (ed.) (1993), *Emmins on Sentencing*, London: Blackstone Press.

Watson, J.P. (1994), 'Too Few Beds', *Psychiatric Bulletin*, 18, 9, p. 531.

Wilding, P. (1990), 'Privatisation: An Introduction and a Critique' in Parry, R. (ed.), *Privatisation*, Research Highlights in Social Work No. 18, London: Jessica Kinglsey Publishers Ltd.

Young, W. (ed.) (1981), *Dangerousness and Criminal Justice*, Howard League for Penal Reform, Cambridge Studies in Criminology: Heinemann.

Young, P. (1988), *The Prison Cell*, London: Adam Smith Institute.

Statutes and Cases

Criminal Appeal Act, 1968.

Criminal Justice Act (Contracted Out Prisons), (No. 2), Order 1992.

Criminal Procedure (Insanity), Act 1964.

Criminal Procedure (Insanity and Fitness to Plead), Act 1991.

Homicide Act 1957.

Mental Health Act 1983.

National Health Service Act 1977.

M'Naghten's Case [1843] 10 Cl & Fin, 200.
R v. Byrne [1960] 2 QB 396.
R v. Gardiner [1967] 1 WLR 464.
R v. Kemp [1957] 1 QB 399.
R v. Sullivan [1983] 3 WLR 123.
X v. United Kingdom [1981] 4 EHRR 181.